EFFECTS OF HEALTH PROGRAMS ON CHILD MORTALITY IN SUB-SAHARAN AFRICA

• • • • • • • • • • • • • • • • • •

Douglas C. Ewbank and James N. Gribble, Editors

Working Group on the Effects of Child Survival and
General Health Programs on Mortality

Panel on the Population Dynamics of Sub-Saharan Africa

Committee on Population

Commission on Behavioral and Social Sciences and Education

National Research Council

NATIONAL ACADEMY PRESS
Washington, D.C.   1993

NATIONAL ACADEMY PRESS • 2101 Constitution Avenue, N.W. • Washington, D.C. 20418

NOTICE: The project that is the subject of this report was approved by the Governing Board of the National Research Council, whose members are drawn from the councils of the National Academy of Sciences, the National Academy of Engineering, and the Institute of Medicine. The members of the committee responsible for the report were chosen for their special competences and with regard for appropriate balance.

This report has been reviewed by a group other than the authors according to procedures approved by a Report Review Committee consisting of members of the National Academy of Sciences, the National Academy of Engineering, and the Institute of Medicine.

The National Academy of Sciences is a private, nonprofit, self-perpetuating society of distinguished scholars engaged in scientific and engineering research, dedicated to the further-ance of science and technology and to their use for the general welfare. Upon the authority of the charter granted to it by the Congress in 1863, the Academy has a mandate that requires it to advise the federal government on scientific and technical matters. Dr. Bruce M. Alberts is president of the National Academy of Sciences.

The National Academy of Engineering was established in 1964, under the charter of the National Academy of Sciences, as a parallel organization of outstanding engineers. It is autonomous in its administration and in the selection of its members, sharing with the National Academy of Sciences the responsibility for advising the federal government. The National Academy of Engineering also sponsors engineering programs aimed at meeting national needs, encourages education and research, and recognizes the superior achievements of engineers. Dr. Robert M. White is president of the National Academy of Engineering.

The Institute of Medicine was established in 1970 by the National Academy of Sciences to secure the services of eminent members of appropriate professions in the examination of policy matters pertaining to the health of the public. The Institute acts under the responsibility given to the National Academy of Sciences by its congressional charter to be an adviser to the federal government and, upon its own initiative, to identify issues of medical care, research, and education. Dr. Kenneth I. Shine is president of the Institute of Medicine.

The National Research Council was organized by the National Academy of Sciences in 1916 to associate the broad community of science and technology with the Academy's pur-poses of furthering knowledge and advising the federal government. Functioning in accor-dance with general policies determined by the Academy, the Council has become the principal operating agency of both the National Academy of Sciences and the National Academy of Engineering in providing services to the government, the public, and the scientific and engi-neering communities. The Council is administered jointly by both Academies and the Institute of Medicine. Dr. Bruce M. Alberts and Dr. Robert M. White are chairman and vice chairman, respectively, of the National Research Council.

Library of Congress Catalog Card No. 93-84761
International Standard Book Number 0-309-04941-5

Additional copies of this report are available from: National Academy Press, 2101 Constitu-tion Avenue, N.W., Box 285, Washington, D.C. 20418. Call 800-624-6242 or 202-334-3313 (in the Washington Metropolitan Area).

B165

---

*through July 1992

Preface

This report is one in a series of studies that have been carried out under the auspices of the Panel on the Population Dynamics of Sub-Saharan Africa of the National Research Council (NRC) Committee on Population. The Research Council has a long history of examining population issues in developing countries. In 1971 it issued the report *Rapid Population Growth: Consequences and Policy Implications.* In 1977, the predecessor Committee on Population and Demography began a major study of levels and trends of fertility and mortality in the developing world that resulted in 13 country reports and 6 reports on demographic methods. Then, in the early 1980s, it undertook a study of the determinants of fertility in the developing world, which resulted in 10 reports. In the mid- and late-1980s, the Committee on Population assessed the economic consequences of population growth and the health consequences of contraceptive use and controlled fertility, among many other activities.

No publication on the demography of sub-Saharan Africa emerged from the early work of the committee, largely because of the paucity of data and the poor quality of what was available. However, censuses, ethnographic studies, and surveys of recent years, such as those under the auspices of the World Fertility Survey and the Demographic and Health Survey programs, have made available data on the demography of sub-Saharan Africa. The data collection has no doubt been stimulated by the increasing interest of both scholars and policymakers in the demographic development of Africa and the relations between demographic change and socioeconomic developments. In response to this interest, the Committee on Population held a meeting in 1989 to ascertain the feasibility and desirability of a major study of the demography of Africa, and decided to set up a Panel on the Population Dynamics of Sub-Saharan Africa.

The panel, which is chaired by Kenneth Hill and includes members from Africa, Europe, and the United States, met for the first time in February 1990 in Washington, D.C. At that meeting the panel decided to set up six working groups, composed of its own members and other experts on the demography of Africa, to carry out specific studies. Four working groups focused on cross-national studies of substantive issues: the social dynamics of adolescent fertility, factors affecting contraceptive use, the effects on mortality of child survival and general health programs, and the demographic effects of economic reversals. The two other working groups were charged with in-depth studies of Kenya and Senegal, with the objective of studying linkages between demographic variables and between those variables and socioeconomic changes. The panel also decided to publish a volume of papers reviewing levels and trends of fertility, nuptiality, the proximate determinants of fertility, child mortality, adult mortality, internal migration, and international migration, as well as the demographic consequences of the AIDS epidemic.

This volume, one of the four cross-national studies, attempts to document the effects of general health and child survival programs on mortality. Although progress has been made, infant and child mortality levels in parts of sub-Saharan Africa remain among the highest in the world. The disease-specific orientation of this report draws attention to a variety of strategies and interventions that have been developed in an effort to reduce the mortality effects of many of the most important diseases. It also examines the effects of general health programs that have been implemented in various settings of sub-Saharan Africa.

As is the case for all of the panel's work, this report would not have been possible without the cooperation and assistance of the Demographic and Health Survey (DHS) Program of the Institute for Resource Development/Macro Systems. We are grateful to the DHS staff for responding to our inquiries and facilitating our early access to the survey data.

We are also grateful to the organizations that provided financial support for the work of the panel: the Office of Health, the Office of Population, and the Africa Bureau of the U.S. Agency for International Development; the Andrew W. Mellon Foundation; the William and Flora Hewlett Foundation; and the Rockefeller Foundation. Besides providing funding, the representatives of these organizations were a source of information and advice in the development of the panel's overall work plan.

This report results from the joint efforts of the working group members and staff and represents a consensus of the members' views on the issues addressed. The Committee on Population and the Panel on the Population Dynamics of Sub-Saharan Africa appreciate the time and energy that all the working group members devoted to the study.

The working group was assisted in its efforts by several commissioned background papers. Charles Katende authored a paper on infant and child mortality and the proximity of health facilities in Liberia and Zimbabwe. Margaret Luck wrote a paper on mortality trends in Senegal.

Special thanks are also due Joan Montgomery Halford and Paula Melville for providing superb administrative and logistical support to the working group and to Florence Poillon for her skillful editing of the report. Eugenia Grohman and Elaine McGarraugh were instrumental in guiding the report through the report review and production processes.

SAMUEL H. PRESTON, *Chair*
Committee on Population

Contents

Executive Summary

Infant and child mortality rates in many parts of sub-Saharan Africa have been decreasing in recent decades, but remain among the highest in the world. Although the decline in mortality is fairly well documented, it has been difficult to determine the relative importance of various diseases and conditions as causes of death among children of different age groups. Data on causes of death are incomplete and of questionable quality, but virtually all studies report that measles, diarrheal diseases, acute respiratory infections, and malaria are the leading causes of death for children less than 5 years of age. This report reviews programs aimed at preventing and treating these and other leading causes of death in sub-Saharan Africa. It also reviews the evidence of the effects of general health programs on reducing child mortality in the region.

Many causes of death can be prevented through vaccination programs. We have reviewed studies of vaccine efficacy and immunization programs in specific locales in sub-Saharan Africa, and have concluded that vaccination programs can have substantial effects on reducing infant and child mortality. However, results from these studies should be extrapolated to different parts of Africa with caution because of ecological and cultural differences, and variations in disease epidemiologies across regions. Moreover, results from small-scale studies are difficult to replicate in large-scale national programs because of differences in program management and logistics.

However, not all the leading causes of death can be prevented through

1

vaccinations. Other diseases responsible for many infant and child deaths can be prevented or treated through a variety of interventions that can be effective if used correctly and in a timely way.

DISEASE- AND INTERVENTION-SPECIFIC FINDINGS

Studies indicate that increased measles vaccination coverage has led to lower mortality. Moreover, the incidence of measles decreases as vaccination coverage increases. Even so, research is needed on appropriate case-management strategies for lowering the case-fatality rates among those who become infected.

Rates of mortality due to diarrheal diseases peak as children are weaned in the postneonatal period. Most interventions in both hospitals and communities focus on case management of acute dehydrating diarrhea by using oral rehydration therapy (ORT) and continued feeding. ORT is an effective treatment, but it is not used widely enough and is often used incorrectly. Research needs include the development and evaluation of home-based treatment programs, the development of case-management strategies for other forms of diarrheal diseases, and an assessment of the effect of ORT programs on mortality.

Malaria is a major health problem in Africa for both children and adults, and is responsible for a large proportion of all child deaths. Programs to combat malaria need to consider the diversity of ecologies, the spread of chloroquine-resistant strains, and the high costs and managerial complexities of many of the available technologies. Presumptive treatment of malaria based on the presence of a fever is common both at clinics and at home, but little research has been done to evaluate the effect of presumptive treatment on mortality. Other increasingly common preventive strategies include providing chemoprophylaxis to pregnant women and the use of insecticide-treated bed nets to prevent mosquito bites.

Acute respiratory infections (ARIs), especially pneumonia, can be treated with antibiotics, but few large-scale studies have been conducted to test different strategies for providing treatment. Those studies that have been conducted suggest that appropriate case management can reduce infant mortality by 20 percent and under-5 mortality by 25 percent. Data from the Demographic and Health Surveys suggest that only a small fraction of children thought to have ARIs actually receive antibiotic treatment.

Other diseases and conditions contributing to infant and child mortality reviewed in this report include pertussis, tuberculosis, tetanus, and nutrition-related conditions.

In addition to the disease-specific interventions that have been initiated in recent years, the expansion of general health services has also contributed to mortality reduction. Studies report declines in mortality as different types of health services become available. The effects of health services on mortality are difficult to evaluate because of timing in implementation and the confounding effects of other factors. Research needs include documenting the effects of primary health care on infant and child mortality, and indicating the factors contributing to its different degrees of success.

GENERAL CONCLUSIONS

In addition to research needs related to specific diseases, this report offers eight observations related to the state of health programs and research in sub-Saharan Africa:

1. Declines in mortality rates should remain the ultimate indicator of the effectiveness of child health interventions in Africa.

2. The goals stated for many programs suggest that program planners often have unrealistic expectations about the feasibility of measuring mortality changes associated with some kinds of interventions. Programs can be classified into three groups: those causing rapid reductions in mortality; those with a more modest potential or that reduce mortality at a slower rate; and those for which direct measurement of mortality effect is not feasible. Misunderstanding the nature of a program can lead to unrealistic expectations of its effects.

3. The trend toward stating program goals in terms of reduction in cause-specific mortality may be setting unrealistic expectations for evaluation.

4. More emphasis should be given to age-specific mortality rates in stating program goals.

5. There is a need for more evaluations of various packages of interventions. It is difficult to evaluate individual components when services are provided in combination.

6. More empirical evaluations of program effects are needed in order to test predictions from models.

7. There is a need for more long-term studies that include regular collection of vital statistics, and routine surveys of service utilization and quality of care.

8. All evaluation studies should include detailed measurement of both the coverage and the promptness of services, as well as compliance with program protocols.

1

Introduction

The historically high population growth rates experienced in Africa were the result of sustained high fertility levels as infant and child mortality began to fall. Recent data from the Demographic and Health Surveys conducted in sub-Saharan Africa indicate that the total fertility rates of a number of countries, most notably Botswana, Kenya, and Zimbabwe, have begun to decrease. Although fertility is declining in these and possibly other parts of sub-Saharan Africa (see Cohen, 1993), it remains high in most of the region. The declines in Botswana, Kenya, and Zimbabwe have been more apparent and rapid than those of other countries in the region.

Similarly, analysis of child mortality trends (i.e., deaths among children under age 5) also suggests that declines are continuing to occur in a number of countries. The rate at which the declines are occurring varies across the region. One of the factors contributing to the decline in infant and child mortality has been the provision of health services. A number of initiatives over the past 25 years have fostered child survival through promoting relatively simple, affordable, and proven technologies.

In 1978, the World Health Assembly set the goal of "health for all by the year 2000." This goal includes ensuring a life both long and free of a heavy burden of illness. In Africa, between 1985 and 1990, an estimated 4.1 million (Heligman et al., 1993) died annually before their fifth birthday and are deprived of the most basic requirements for a healthy life. Therefore, the first aim of many health programs in Africa is to provide children with a reasonable chance of living a long and healthy life.

This emphasis on lowering mortality is also evident in the U.S. Agency for International Development's (USAID) Child Survival Initiative, which started in Africa in 1985. The program's goal is to reduce infant mortality in USAID-supported countries from the 1985 average of 97 death per 1,000 live births to less than 75. The program builds on primary health care programs, and focuses on immunizations, oral rehydration therapy, improving nutrition, reducing numbers of high-risk births, and improving maternal health. Since 1985, USAID has invested U.S. $1.5 billion in the Child Survival Initiative.

In September 1990 at the World Summit for Children, representatives of 159 countries agreed on a Plan of Action for Implementing the World Declaration on the Survival, Protection and Development of Children in the 1990s. The plan includes seven major goals, the first of which is targeted to be completed between 1990 and the year 2000: a reduction of infant and under-5 mortality rates by one-third, or to 50 and 70 per 1,000 live births, respectively, whichever is less (United Nations Children's Fund, 1991).

Among the more specific supporting goals were the elimination of neonatal tetanus by 1995 and the reduction of measles deaths by 95 percent by the year 2000, as well as the reduction of deaths due to diarrhea in children less than 5 years of age by 50 percent, and the reduction of deaths due to acute respiratory infections in children under 5 by one-third (United Nations Children's Fund, 1991). The plan included many other goals for child health: for example, increasing birthweights and reducing the prevalence of malnutrition, and of iodine and vitamin A deficiencies. However, reduction of child mortality is the major element of the goals for child health.

Although infant and child mortality rates are declining in most of sub-Saharan Africa, only two countries—Botswana and Zimbabwe—currently are estimated to have infant and child mortality rates as low as the major goal calls for by the year 2000. Most other countries will require declines of more than one-third to achieve the goals of infant mortality rates of 50 per 1,000 and child mortality rates of 70 per 1,000. In the past, mortality reductions probably have been the result of a number of different factors, including health programs (and control of epidemics), changes in diets and health behaviors, and general economic development visible in education and road building, among others. These factors will all continue to play a role in reducing mortality in the future. However, the most direct way in which governments can intervene to reduce mortality in the short run is through increased provision of health services.

The ability of African governments to provide health services is limited by the small amount of money available for the health sector. Half of the population of Africa lives in countries where expenditures on health were in the range of $1.50 to $6.80 per capita in 1985. The average African lives in a country in which the government expenditure on health was only $5.32

per person (United Nations Children's Fund, 1991; Ogbu and Gallagher, 1992). Between 1975 and 1985, the average African experienced a decline of 11 percent in the government's real per capita expenditures on health.

The severe shortage of funds for health programs has led to a debate about the best strategy for developing health services. Although there are many dimensions to this debate, the central argument has been between those advocating "selective" primary health care and those advocating "comprehensive" primary health care. (See, for example, Walsh and Warren, 1979; Habicht and Berman, 1980; Newell, 1988, for more discussion.)

The advocates of a selective approach argue that the shortage of resources requires that efforts be focused on the most cost-effective interventions. The advocates of a comprehensive approach argue that relying on cost-effectiveness leads to a short-term strategy that will make it difficult to reach the long-term goal. In particular, they argue that the most cost-effective programs are often individual programs aimed at selected health problems, for example, vaccination-preventable diseases and malaria control. However, if too much emphasis is placed on vertically organized intervention-specific, the goal of integrated programs may never be achieved, and only a limited number of services will be available to the general public.

Whether programs are integrated or not, the severe financial constraints on health programs in Africa require choices, such as which drugs to purchase and which skills to emphasize in training health personnel, among others. Without massive increases in the funds available for health programs, African governments will have to set priorities (implicit or explicit) for the use of scarce resources. In addition to cost-effectiveness, there are many other criteria for setting these priorities, including costs, efficacy, concerns for equity, and the preferences of the population. Given the goals set by the World Summit for Children and the high mortality rates in Africa, it seems initially reasonable to stress the expected effect of programs on mortality.

Comparing programs according to their expected effect on mortality has several advantages. First, mortality rates provide a common measure that facilitates comparison of programs. For example, mortality rates allow us to compare the effect of a measles vaccination program with the effect of a program for treating diarrhea. Second, reductions in mortality often reflect reductions in the duration or severity of illnesses. For example, a program that treats or prevents malaria may lower mortality by reducing the incidence, prevalence, or severity of malaria. It is difficult to produce a simple measure of morbidity that incorporates both prevalence and severity. However, if mortality due to infectious diseases can be reduced through a program, it is likely that morbidity also declines.

It is not feasible to measure the mortality effect of every health program in every country. However, it is important to measure the mortality effect of various types of interventions. When we know that a specific type of program can reduce mortality, we can reasonably assume that any similar program that reaches a substantial proportion of the population with quality services probably reduces mortality.

This volume examines the scientific evidence of the effectiveness of a variety of health interventions in reducing child mortality in sub-Saharan Africa. We have not evaluated the expected effect of potential new technologies yet to be tried in Africa, such as vaccines to protect against malaria or AIDS. We have also limited the review to interventions that are generally the province of health ministries. For example, we have not evaluated the impact of water and sanitation programs, agricultural projects, or adult literacy programs, although these might be important components of government strategies for reducing child mortality. For the majority of these types of programs, there is little evidence of a mortality effect. In addition, we have limited ourselves to programs whose effect on mortality can be evaluated. For this reason we have not evaluated the evidence on AIDS programs. The delay between human immunodeficiency virus (HIV) infection and death is so long that it is not feasible to measure directly the effect of programs on mortality.

We have limited the scope of this report to the demographic and epidemiologic evidence that programs have reduced mortality. This focus provides only half of the evidence needed to carry out a ranking of programs in terms of cost-effectiveness. However, by limiting our review to programs that are already common in Africa, we have focused on programs that are generally assumed to be cost-effective. This review examines whether the evidence of effectiveness justifies the common perception that these programs are effective. It would be useful to determine whether studies of the costs of these programs (including both public and private costs) justify the usual perceptions. However, a complete review of cost studies would extend beyond the resources and the technical expertise of the working group.

In evaluating the mortality effect of health interventions, we go beyond the evidence that these technologies are "safe and effective." Health programs do not include medical technologies unless there is evidence that their medical benefits outweigh the medical risks for individuals. We are interested in the benefits to populations, and these can be very different from the benefits to individuals. In the terms of evaluation studies, we need to go beyond estimating intervention "efficacy," the biological effect as measured in carefully controlled clinical trials. Instead we need to measure the "effectiveness" of programs, which can be reduced by improper procedures, low compliance rates, or factors that select individuals who receive treatment. For example, programs to prevent measles, malaria, or tuberculosis can change the epidemiology of the disease by changing the risk of infection for the entire population, including those not receiving treatment.

Decision makers should be aware of the differences in results based on biological models and those from field studies. Theoretical results based on models rarely serve as a substitute for field studies, which incorporate the difficulties and shortcomings arising in carrying out a program.

Often, the field-based evidence that health interventions reduce mortality rates is weak. The justification for many programs is based on the argument that a given disease causes death in a certain percentage of cases, and that the intervention is effective at a certain level in preventing (or curing) the disease and has few or no side effects. These arguments rely on biological models of the disease process and scientific tests of various parts of the model (e.g., the efficacy of a vaccine or treatment). This approach is most convincing when the evidence suggests very few serious side effects and when the disease has serious implications for health (e.g., the use of measles vaccination).

The evidence to support these biological models may not be adequate to produce reliable population-based estimates of program effectiveness. For example, many of the deaths of children in Africa result from the interaction of several health problems. It is difficult, if not impossible, to design models that describe these interactions in sufficient detail to produce reliable estimates for the mortality-reducing effect of different types of programs.

Estimating the effect of a health intervention becomes more difficult when the program does not reach all children at risk for the disease. For example, a program that reaches children only in the upper socioeconomic groups will probably have less effect on mortality than one that targets malnourished children in impoverished families. As a result of the unequal distribution of risks, there can be large differences in the effectiveness of programs that employ the same medical technologies. For this reason, we must examine the effectiveness of programs in a number of different settings, not just the potential efficacy of technologies.

Much of the evidence about the effectiveness of interventions on mortality comes from research projects in small populations. Thus, the evidence from these projects may not provide reasonable estimates of the effects these interventions will have when implemented in large-scale government programs. When programs are expanded beyond small populations, the quality of the services can change drastically as can the social groups they reach. Vaccine failures, incorrect diagnoses, and reduced effectiveness of supervision or patient education are all more likely in large-scale programs.

This volume begins with a discussion of mortality trends and levels over the past three decades in the region. Mortality has decreased in all parts of Africa, but at varying rates, as illustrated by regional differentials.

The cause-of-death profile varies across areas, but a small number of diseases accounts for most of the infant and child mortality throughout the region. However, because data are generally of poor quality or nonexistent, it is difficult to rank these specific diseases.

Most of this volume examines various types of health programs. Chapters 3, 4, and 5 review evidence on the effectiveness of interventions aimed at individual diseases. Chapter 3 examines the diseases that can be prevented or reduced by immunization: measles, pertussis, tuberculosis, leprosy, and tetanus. Chapter 4 focuses on interventions targeted at other communicable diseases: diarrheal diseases, malaria, and acute respiratory infections. Nutritional conditions, including protein-energy malnutrition, low birthweight, and vitamin A deficiency are discussed in Chapter 5. The discussions of these specific diseases and conditions examine the etiology, symptoms, and prevalence of each disease; its epidemiology and natural course; intervention studies conducted in Africa and other parts of the world; and program coverage in Africa.

The organization of the bulk of the report by disease reflects the fact that almost all of the studies of the effectiveness of health programs examine single interventions. Although we would have preferred to organize the report along other lines, the available research does not support other approaches. In particular, there is very little research on the effectiveness of the most common type of programs, namely those programs that combine interventions against several diseases. What evidence there is on the effectiveness of integrated and general health programs is reviewed in Chapter 6. The final chapter provides conclusions and recommendations.

2

Trends in Mortality and Causes of Death in Africa

During the past 30 years, African governments have worked to increase the quantity and quality of modern health services available to their populations. Before independence, most colonial governments introduced health programs. If the expansion of health services has had an effect, we should expect to find that infant and child mortality has declined during recent decades, at least in countries that have achieved improvements in services. Of course, there have been numerous other changes in Africa that might have contributed to mortality reduction. Increasing education levels are associated with improved child care practices and better utilization of health services. Construction of roads reduces the effect of droughts by improving food distribution networks. Moreover, road construction facilitates transportation to urban areas where more modern health services are located.

This chapter reviews data collection and techniques for estimating trends, mortality levels and trends, verbal autopsies, causes of death, and the effect of AIDS on child mortality. The discussions of mortality levels and causes of death provide the background for later chapters, which consider the evidence for the effects of specific programs.

TRENDS IN CHILD MORTALITY

Data Collection and Estimation Techniques

Early attempts to measure mortality levels of African populations were based on efforts to register all births and deaths, especially in urban areas.

For instance, a vital registration system was implemented as early as 1915 in four cities of Senegal and continues to be maintained. Despite many attempts, the coverage and quality of vital registration systems remain poor at the national level in continental sub-Saharan Africa (De Graft-Johnson, 1988).

Most recent efforts to estimate mortality levels and trends at the national level are based on large-scale surveys and censuses. These surveys employ two basic approaches to estimating infant and child mortality. The first approach involves direct methods, which are based on reported births and deaths of individual children. The most common survey approach is the maternity history, which includes the date of each birth and the date or age at death of each child who has died. Maternity histories have formed the core of both the World Fertility Surveys (WFS) and the Demographic and Health Surveys (DHS). Variations include truncated maternity histories, which include only recent births (i.e., children born during the past five years or the two most recent children born to each mother). Death rates can be calculated directly from these data because they allow tabulations of deaths and person-years of risk at each age. Trends in mortality can be estimated from tabulation of deaths and person-years of risk by both age and year. A second type of direct estimation procedure is based on information about recent deaths (generally deaths in the last year) and the current population size.

The alternative approach is to use indirect methods, which are based on data that do not provide for tabulation of deaths and person-years of risk by age. The most common indirect approach is the Brass child survival method, which uses data on the average numbers of children ever born and the surviving children of women in each five-year age group, along with a simple model. This model requires assumptions about the age pattern of child mortality. It can be used to estimate trends in mortality on the further assumption that the trends in recent years have been smooth. Several variants of this model are described in detail in United Nations Manual X (United Nations Department of International Economic and Social Affairs, 1983).

Most of the data on levels and trends come from comparisons of several surveys in the same country. When a country has a consistent combination of estimates of levels and trends from direct and indirect methods, the statistical evidence can be considered reliable. However, Hill (1992) recently reviewed the available data from 38 sub-Saharan African countries and found as many cases of inconsistent as of consistent data. Common shortcomings of data on child survival include the omission and displacement of births and deaths and misreporting of ages and durations of exposure to the risk of death. Although the general impression of mortality decline is strong, the estimated trends should be considered with caution because of these types of error in data.

In addition to national data, more accurate local studies can provide detailed information and a check on the plausibility of national data. Examples include some of the vital registration systems of cities and some prospective studies of communities. In these research areas with continuous registration of vital events, a small, geographically defined community is followed for a period of time with a multiround survey—the frequency of which can range from weekly to annually—and periodic censuses. These intensive undertakings provide complete and accurate demographic data, including trends, age patterns, seasonal variations, differentials, and sometimes, causes of death, though typically for fairly small numbers of events.

Current Levels of Mortality and Trends Since 1960

The measure we use for tracking levels and trends of child mortality is the probability of dying by age 5 ($_5q_0$), expressed per thousand live births. This measure captures almost all the mortality risk prior to adulthood, and is less affected by the age profile of child rearing practices such as weaning than the infant mortality rate. Estimates of $_5q_0$ are available after 1980 for 15 of 39 sub-Saharan African countries. Table 2-1 presents the probability of dying by age 5 for the years before 1960 to 1985 for all the countries of sub-Saharan Africa with acceptable estimates. The number of estimates for each year ranges from 15 (for 1985) to 27 (for 1970). The recent estimates vary from 100 or fewer deaths by age 5 per 1,000 live births in Botswana, Kenya, and Zimbabwe to 200 or more in Burkina Faso, Liberia, Mali, and Zaire. The remaining countries cluster around 160. The low-mortality countries have mortality rates comparable to those in many countries of Asia, with levels lower than India or Pakistan. The high-mortality countries include the highest values of child mortality recorded in the world during the 1980s.

The data for almost all African countries show declining mortality since 1960. Figure 2-1 shows data from Table 2-1, with different symbols used for data points from the broad subregions—western, middle, eastern, and southern. Three points stand out from Figure 2-1. First, there is a great deal of variability in measures of child mortality among countries of sub-Saharan Africa. In 1960, probabilities of dying by age 5 varied from 140 to 400 among the 19 countries with estimates; in 1985, the range was from 60 to 250 across the 15 countries with estimates. Second, there has been a substantial and rather steady decline in child mortality risks from 1960 to 1985; the median $_5q_0$ in 1960 of 225 fell to 180 by 1985. Third, there is a substantial differential in child mortality between the countries of eastern and southern Africa and those of middle and western Africa; although affected by the countries included in the data set for specific years, the median $_5q_0$ values for eastern and southern Africa are about 60 per thousand lower than those for western and middle Africa from 1960 to 1985.

TABLE 2-1   Child Mortality Rates per 1,000 Live Births (based on the probability of dying by age 5), by Country and Year, Pre-1960 Through 1985

Country	Pre-1960	1960	1965	1970	1975	1980	1985
Eastern Africa							
Burundi	—	270	240	220	220	210	175
Ethiopia	—	235	230	225	220	—	—
Kenya	260	210	185	165	145	125	100
Malawi	—	360	345	335	320	285	—
Mozambique	260	—	280	280	280	—	—
Rwanda	—	240	220	220	220	220	—
Somalia	—	—	240	225	210	—	—
Tanzania	260	240	235	225	215	—	—
Uganda	245	225	195	180	175	185	185
Zambia	—	220	190	180	165	150	—
Zimbabwe	—	160	155	145	140	135	95
Middle Africa							
Angola	360	—	—	—	—	—	—
Cameroon	290	—	235	220	185	—	—
Central African Republic	—	325	295	245	—	—	—
Chad	340	310	—	—	—	—	—
Congo	290	200	165	140	—	—	—
Equatorial Guinea	—	—	—	—	—	—	—
Gabon	350	250	—	—	—	—	—
Zaire	285	—	—	—	235	210	200
Southern Africa							
Botswana	—	175	160	140	120	90	60
Lesotho	—	200	195	185	175	—	—
Namibia	—	—	—	—	—	—	—
South Africa	—	—	—	—	—	—	—
Swaziland	240	230	220	215	—	—	—
Western Africa							
Benin	360	—	—	255	240	200	—
Burkina Faso	420	315	295	275	255	220	215
Côte d'Ivoire	—	—	265	245	210	165	140
The Gambia	—	350	345	310	275	240	—
Ghana	370	220	210	185	170	155	160
Guinea	380	—	—	—	—	—	—
Guinea-Bissau	300	—	—	—	—	—	—
Liberia	—	280	270	255	245	235	220
Mali	385	—	—	—	360	310	250
Niger	300	—	—	—	—	—	—
Nigeria	—	—	—	—	—	195	190
Senegal	375	300	295	285	265	220	190
Sierra Leone	—	400	385	365	—	—	—
Togo	350	300	245	220	200	180	160
Northern Africa							
Sudan	—	220	205	170	150	145	135

SOURCE: Hill (1992).

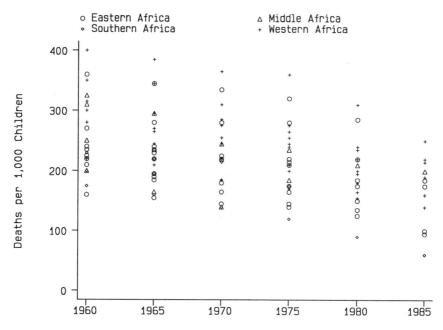

FIGURE 2-1 Estimates of the probability of dying by age 5 ($_5q_0$) by subregion and time period. NOTE: Western Africa (shown as a plus) includes Benin, Burkina Faso, The Gambia, Ghana, Guinea, Guinea-Bissau, Liberia, Mali, Niger, Nigeria, Senegal, Sierra Leone, and Togo. Middle Africa (shown as a triangle) includes Angola, Cameroon, Central African Republic, Chad, Congo, Equitorial Guinea, Gabon, and Zaire. Eastern Africa (shown as a circle) includes Burundi, Ethiopia, Kenya, Malawi, Mozambique, Rwanda, Somalia, Tanzania, Uganda, Zambia, and Zimbabwe. Southern Africa (shown as a diamond) includes Botswana, Lesotho, Namibia, South Africa, and Swaziland. SOURCE: Hill (1992).

In countries where long-term series are available, there is consistent evidence that the mortality decline started well before 1960. A number of estimates of child mortality suggest that current levels reflect long-term, substantial changes. The earliest estimate of $_5q_0$ for Kenya, for example, goes back to 1947, when it was 262 (Hill, 1991). By 1970, the probability of dying before age 5 had decreased to 165, and it was estimated to be 100 by 1985. The estimate of $_5q_0$ for Ghana in 1935 was 371 (Hill, 1991), had declined to 185 by 1970, and continued to decline, although more slowly to 160 in 1985. Senegal also shows a large decrease in mortality, although current levels remain fairly high. The probability of dying by age 5 was estimated to be 373 in 1946 (Hill, 1991); it fell to 285 in 1970, and was estimated to be 190 in 1985. Vital statistics for Dakar, Senegal, suggest that mortality has been declining for at least 70 years.

In general the decline in mortality has been steady since 1960 in most countries. However, exceptions exist. One exception is Ethiopia, with no evidence of decline between 1960 and 1975, and no data thereafter. In Ghana, the decline seems to have stopped after 1980 and there may actually have been some increase. The same seems to be true in Uganda, where mortality appears to have been rising slightly since 1975. The scanty data from Mozambique do not show any evidence of decline. It also appears that mortality did not change in Rwanda between 1960 and 1980. Several of these countries went through periods of major political turmoil during the 1970s and the 1980s.

In several countries, periods for which data are available are too short to permit any serious conclusion about trends. In Nigeria, data are so poor before the 1990 DHS that mortality trends cannot be determined. Other countries—Angola, Chad, and Mauritania—do not have nationally representative data that allow any estimation of mortality.

In addition to variations between countries, there are major variations in mortality levels within countries. These striking subnational differences were noted especially in Kenya, Angola, Niger, and Mozambique by Coale and Lorimer (1967). Large differences were also found by Ewbank et al. (1986) in Kenya. Hill (1992) found variations by district ranging from 140 to 380 in the 1955-1957 survey in Zaire and variations from 130 to 290 in the 1969 census of Zambia. Cantrelle et al. (1986) found large variations in Senegal. Farah and Preston (1982) showed major differences between northern and southern Sudan. Extreme regional differences seem to be a distinctive feature of African mortality, probably reflecting major differences in local epidemiological and socioeconomic environments.

In summary, there is clear evidence that mortality of children under 5 has been declining rapidly in sub-Saharan Africa, in some parts at least since the 1940s and possibly since the 1910s. However, the data are not detailed or precise enough to show the specific effects of health systems and health interventions. Such a conclusion is limited by both the imprecision of the estimated trends in mortality and the difficulty of establishing changes in the quantity and quality of medical services actually provided during each time period, as discussed in Chapter 6. Nonetheless, the mortality decline accompanied the emergence of modern medicine, and the arrival of antibiotics and antimalarial drugs, as well as socioeconomic development, characterized by modern transportation, increase in agricultural and industrial production, urbanization, and modern education.

The extent of political and economic organization in a country seems to play a major role in mortality reduction. Countries where political unrest, war, and famine disrupt the social organization tend to have a stagnant mortality and, in some cases, rising mortality rates. Most likely, future trends in mortality will also continue to be shaped by the combination of improved health services, activities related to economic development, and unexpected social and political problems.

CAUSES OF DEATH AMONG AFRICAN CHILDREN

Information about the major causes of death is important for program planning and can be useful for program evaluation. Programs that target a small number of diseases can use reliable information about changes in the causes of death to demonstrate a causal relationship between program inputs and mortality decline.

Unfortunately, even less is known about the causes of death in Africa than about mortality levels and trends. None of the countries of continental sub-Saharan Africa has a reliable national system of death registration.

In addition, knowledge of causes of death is hampered by two other difficulties. The first problem arises from the fact that many deaths have multiple causes. Consider, for example, a child who is moderately malnourished, has a case of measles, and dies shortly afterward from acute diarrhea and pneumonia. The death could be attributed to any one of these conditions. All of them can be either prevented or treated by appropriate medical interventions. Therefore, the effect of child survival programs on mortality will be determined by the nature of the interaction among these causes. However, the complexity of the disease process is difficult to summarize in simple statistical or tabular form. A cause-of-death classification is reductionist by necessity.

A second problem is the quality of the diagnoses. Even in the best hospitals of Europe and the United States, a number of deaths are assigned to incorrect causes. In developing countries, accurate diagnoses are even more difficult to obtain. One reason is that a large proportion of deaths occur outside modern medical facilities and are not observed by qualified diagnosticians. Even in hospitals, diagnosis is complicated by the lack of complete and accurate case histories, a low rate of autopsy, and a shortage of diagnostic facilities. In addition, many patients arrive at the hospital during the last stages of the disease, which makes it difficult to disentangle the proximate causes. This situation inhibits a clearer understanding of the role of malnutrition in morbidity and mortality.

Verbal Autopsies

A number of researchers have used a technique called "verbal autopsy" to assess the causes of deaths that were not attended by trained medical personnel (e.g., Garenne and Fontaine, 1986; Gray et al., 1990). The concept behind this technique is to use all the available evidence—clinical, epidemiological, and demographic—to determine the probable causes of death. Although verbal autopsies provide guesses of the causes of deaths that might otherwise have been included in a miscellaneous category of "other deaths," these gains can be illusory. In particular, verbal autopsies, like all diagnostic techniques, can lead to false attribution. In some cases, these false positives may outnumber the true cases.

Little is known about the precision of algorithms (i.e., the series of questions asked to determine the cause of death) used in verbal autopsies. For example, what is the ability of algorithms for malaria to pick up all cases of malaria (i.e., the sensitivity of the algorithm, denoted here by α) or their ability to identify deaths due to other causes as "nonmalarial" (i.e., the specificity, β)? Given the limited amount and types of information that can be collected in a verbal autopsy, it is difficult to achieve high rates of both sensitivity and specificity. If the specificity is low and the condition is rare, then the estimated proportion of deaths due to a cause is likely to be exaggerated. On the other hand if the sensitivity is low and the condition is common, the estimated rate might be understated.

Kalter et al. (1990) studied some algorithms for tetanus, measles, diarrhea, and acute lower respiratory infections (ALRI) in the Philippines. Table 2-2 presents their results for four sets of criteria for diagnosing ALRI. As expected, the specificity of algorithms increased with the number of items included in the algorithm, but the sensitivity declined accordingly. Thus, with more symptoms, fewer cases of ALRI were picked up, but those that were detected were more likely to be real cases (i.e., an increased positive predictive value).

TABLE 2-2   Sensitivity and Specificity of Various
Criteria for Diagnosing Acute Lower Respiratory
Infections in the Phillipines

Criteria	Sensitivity α (%)	Specificity β (%)
A. Cough and dyspnea	86	47
B. Cough and dyspnea ≥1 day	66	60
C. Cough ≥4 days and dyspnea ≥1 day	59	77
D. Cough ≥4 days and dyspnea ≥2 days	41	93

SOURCE: Kalter et al. (1990:384). By permission of Oxford University Press.

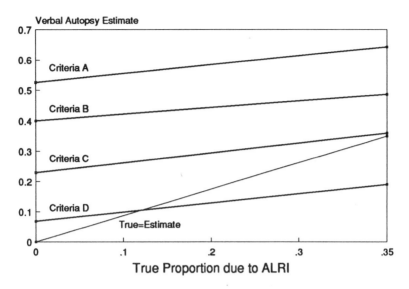

FIGURE 2-2 Relationship between true proportion of deaths to acute lower respiratory infection and proportion estimated from verbal autopsies using four sets of criteria for diagnosis.

The implications of this trade-off between sensitivity and specificity for the estimated proportion of deaths due to ALRI are shown in Figure 2-2. If the real proportion of deaths due to this cause is ρ, and the sensitivity and specificity of the diagnostic criteria are α and β, then the estimated proportion of deaths due to the cause is $\alpha\rho + (1 - \beta)(1 - \rho)$. For example, if ALRI was not responsible for any deaths in a population, criteria C (cough of four or more days and breathing difficulty of one or more days) would still estimate that 23 percent were due to ALRI because the specificity of these criteria is only 77 percent. If 35 percent of the deaths are truly caused by ALRI, then the false diagnoses of ALRI by using criteria C are counterbalanced by missed cases of ALRI. In this case the estimated proportion of deaths due to ALRI is 36 percent, which is very close to the true 35 percent.

Criteria D (cough of four or more days and breathing difficulty of two or more days) have a higher specificity (and lower sensitivity), and produce an accurate estimate if ALRI is actually responsible for 10 percent of deaths. If ALRI is responsible for more than 10 percent, criteria D underestimate the true rate. If ALRI is responsible for less than 10 percent, criteria D lead to an overestimate. Criteria A (cough and breathing difficulty) and B (cough and breathing difficulty of one or more days) have such low specificities (47 and 60 percent, respectively) that they do not produce reasonable estimates of the proportion of deaths due to ALRI at any plausible true level.

Reasonable estimates of the proportion of deaths due to ALRI (or any other cause that is responsible for less than 30 percent of deaths in an age group) are obtained only if the specificity of the criteria is quite high. For example, with a sensitivity of 65 percent and a specificity of 80 percent, the prevalence of a cause that is actually responsible for 15 percent of deaths will be overestimated by 78 percent (i.e., it will be estimated to be 27 percent of deaths). In some cases, it may not be possible to achieve levels of specificity high enough for important causes of child deaths in Africa.

Snow et al. (1992) used verbal autopsies for 303 infants who died at Kilifi hospital in Kenya. However, Becker and Gray (personal communication) have raised several questions about the questionnaire used by Snow et al. They note in particular that measles, accidents, and malnutrition are the only causes that were addressed by specific items in the questionnaire. All other diagnoses apparently were based on responses to a checklist of 29 symptoms and signs. It is not clear how the interviewers asked the questions on the checklist, and it is not known what algorithms were used to derive the verbal autopsy diagnoses. Because of these problems, the results obtained by Snow et al. do not necessarily reflect the sensitivities and specificities that could be achieved by the type of detailed questionnaires and algorithms used in other studies. Therefore, the study by Snow et al. does not provide a test of the true potential of verbal autopsies.

Mobley et al. (personal communication, 1993) examined the sensitivity and specificity of carefully defined algorithms for five major causes of death in Namibia. Their sample included deaths in a hospital of children who were diagnosed with malnutrition, diarrhea, pneumonia, malaria or measles either at the time of admission or before the time of death. Sixty-one percent of the cases had two or more of these diagnoses.

Mobley et al. (personal communication, 1993) reviewed the reliability of several algorithms for each disease. For diarrhea deaths, the presence of loose or liquid stool combined with either thirst or sunken eyes gave a sensitivity of 75 percent and a specificity of 71 percent. Raising the specificity to 90 percent by using only the presence of 6 or more loose or liquid stools per day leads to a sharp reduction in the sensitivity to 36 percent. For pneumonia, the specificity never rose above 71 percent using the presence of cough and fever combined with difficult or rapid breathing. This algorithm was associated with a sensitivity of only 61 percent. A diagnosis of measles based on age greater than 120 days and rash led to a sensitivity of 71 percent and a specificity of 85 percent. Adding fever for at least three days raised the specificity to 90 percent but dropped the sensitivity to 67 percent. Their algorithms for malaria reached relatively high levels of specificity (several in the range of 87 to 97 percent) based on fever plus convulsions and/or loss of consciousness. However, these were associated with low sensitivities (41 to 45 percent). These algorithms performed better for children diagnosed in the hospital with cerebral malaria.

The above study provides very useful information about the reliability of verbal autopsy estimates for major causes of child mortality in Africa. However, by limiting the sample to deaths ascribed to these five causes in the hospital, the estimated specificities might be different than they would be in a completely random sample of deaths. For example, the specificities for cerebral malaria might have been lower if they had included deaths to meningitis and other infectious diseases that can be associated with high fever and convulsions. However, the fact that even the most stringent algorithms rarely lead to specificities as high as 90 percent suggests that verbal autopsies will rarely be useful for measuring mortality rates for causes of death that are responsible for less than 15 percent of all deaths in an age group.

Studies of Causes of Death Among Infants and Children

The appendix to this volume reviews the results of studies of causes of deaths among infants and children in 9 areas of Africa. These studies are summarized in Table 2-3. Given the problems discussed above, we have to exercise caution in interpreting the results of these studies and in trying to generalize to the whole of sub-Saharan Africa.

Low birthweight, birth trauma, and congenital defects are responsible for the largest number of neonatal deaths in most studies. The few exceptions (western Sierra Leone and Niakhar, Senegal) have very high rates due to neonatal tetanus. During the postneonatal period, diarrheal diseases are generally ranked first, followed by ALRI-pneumonia, malaria, and measles in varying orders.

At ages 1 to 4 years, measles is often the most common cause of death. In some parts of the continent, measles vaccination rates may have increased sufficiently to reduce its importance; however, it certainly continues to be a major factor in child mortality and must remain a top priority for health programs. Diarrheal diseases are generally the second cause of deaths in this age group, with malaria, malnutrition, and ALRI-pneumonia generally ranked third through fifth in varying orders. Of course, it is often difficult to determine a specific cause of death because of the common simultaneous occurrence of measles, ALRI, and diarrhea.

Although it is not possible to produce reliable estimates of the proportions of infant and child deaths in Africa that are due to each major cause, the primary importance of diarrheal diseases, measles, malaria, ARI, and malnutrition is clear. The list can be rounded out with the addition of a few neonatal causes (prematurity, birth trauma, congenital defects, and neonatal tetanus), and the possible addition of a few causes that are more difficult to

TABLE 2-3 Summary of Cause-of-Death Studies by Rank of Importance of Cause

Neonates

Study Area	Tetanus	Low Birthweight	Birth Trauma	Congenital Defect	Pneumonia	Sepsis
Sierra	1	2		4		3
Machakos		1[a]	1[a]	2		
Dakar		1[a]	1[a]	1[a]		
Saint-Louis		1[a]	1[a]	1[a]		
Niakhar	1	2	3	5	4	

Postneonates

Study Area	Diarrhea	ALRI/Pneumonia	Malaria	Measles	Meningitis	Malnutrition	Septicemia
Sierra	2	1	5	3		4	
Machakos	1	2		3			6
Dakar	1	4		2		3	
Saint-Louis	3			2		1	
Bamako	1	6	2	3	4	5	
Malumfashi	2		1	3			
Sudan	1	4		3			
Kasongo	2	1	2				
Niakhar	1	2	3	4		5	

Children 1-4 Years

Study Area	Diarrhea	ALRI/Pneumonia	Malaria	Measles	Meningitis	Malnutrition	Tuberculosis	Accidents
Sierra	4	2	5	1	7	3	6	8
Machakos	3	4		1		2		
Dakar	2	3	4	1				
Saint-Louis	3	5	4	1		2		
Barnako	4	5	2		6	3		
Malumfashi	2		1	3				
Sudan	1	4	3	2				
Kasongo	2	3						
Niakhar	1	2	3	4		5		

[a]These causes ranked equally in the study.

SOURCES: Sudanese Ministry of Health and World Health Organization (1981); Cantrelle et al. (1986); Ewbank et al. (1986); Kandeh (1986); Fargues and Nassour (1988); van Lerberghe and Pangu (1988); Garenne and Fontaine (1990); Omondi-Odhiambo et al. (1990); Tomkins et al. (1991); M. Garenne, personal communication (1992).

diagnose (e.g., pertussis and meningitis). The relative importance of these main causes will vary across populations because of differences in ecology (e.g., malaria), behavior (e.g., neonatal tetanus), and vaccination patterns (e.g., measles). Given the difficulty in determining specific causes of death, it may be unrealistic to determine whether or not the disease-specific reductions in mortality, such as those stated in the goals of the World Summit for Children, are actually being achieved.

Effects of AIDS on Child Mortality

The acquired immune deficiency syndrome epidemic is a new factor influencing infant and child mortality in sub-Saharan Africa. Currently, we do not have solid data on the incidence of AIDS deaths among children in the region. However, we do know that the AIDS epidemic will have both direct and indirect effects on infant and child mortality. The direct transmission of the human immunodeficiency virus (HIV), which causes AIDS, from mother to child occurs primarily during delivery, but may occur also through breast milk. It is estimated that at least 80 percent of children infected with HIV will die by age 5. The indirect effect is the additional mortality risk arising from orphanhood faced by an uninfected child whose mother is ill from or dies of AIDS.

How large are these effects likely to be? Stoto (1993) reviews simulation models of AIDS and finds that infant mortality rates might increase by as much as 20 percent in urban areas. However, these estimates have wide margins of uncertainty. First, the estimates depend critically on perinatal HIV transmission rates. The models assume that about 30 percent of children born to HIV-positive mothers will themselves be HIV positive, although some European studies have shown rates as low as 13.9 percent (European Collaborative Study, 1991). Second, it is not known if HIV-positive women have higher or lower fertility rates than women in general because of social behavior or health status. Third, the estimates consider only the direct effect described above; they do not include the additional risks to AIDS orphans. Such risks may be large for very young children, but probably fall rapidly as age of the child increases.

Simple calculations provide an estimate of the order of magnitude of the effect of AIDS on child mortality in Africa. It is estimated that approximately 2.5 percent of adults in sub-Saharan Africa are HIV positive (U.S. Agency for International Development, 1991). If HIV-positive women have the same fertility rates as other women, then about 2.5 percent of all births in sub-Saharan Africa are to HIV-positive mothers. If the transmission rate from mother to child is 30 percent, and if 80 percent of HIV-infected children die by age 5, then .006 (i.e., .025 • .3 • .8) of children born in Africa will die by age 5 of AIDS. However, about 18 percent of these children would have died by age 5 in the absence of AIDS. Thus, the direct effect of AIDS is to increase mortality by age 5 by about .006 (1 - .18), or 5 per 1,000. Therefore, AIDS is probably responsible for only about 3 percent of all deaths to infants and children in Africa. Adding to this the extra child deaths resulting from orphanhood among HIV-negative children born to HIV-positive mothers would increase this percentage only slightly.

Estimates of the recent effects of AIDS on child mortality in sub-Saharan Africa are uncertain enough; forecasts of its effects for the rest of the decade are more hazardous still. Perinatal transmission rates and case-fatality rates are not likely to change much in the next decade. However, seroprevalence might continue to increase or might start to fall as behavioral modifications occur and high-risk groups are reduced by excess mortality.

SUMMARY

Mortality in virtually all areas of Africa appears to have been declining in recent decades, although the pace of decline has varied greatly. Reductions in infant and child mortality continue to be observed in most countries, although it appears that slight increases have occurred in some countries in recent years. The limited data available indicate that the leading causes of death during the neonatal period are birth trauma, prematurity, and congenital defects, although tetanus was the leading cause of death in a few studies. In the postneonatal period, diarrhea appears to be the leading cause of death, followed by ALRI-pneumonia. Among children ages 1-4 years, measles, diarrhea, ALRI, malaria, and malnutrition are the leading causes of death. Although AIDS is an important cause of deaths among adults in Africa, its effect among infants and children is not large relative to other causes. The transmission of AIDS from mother to infant probably increases infant and child mortality by fewer than 5 deaths per 1,000.

3

Immunization Programs

The Expanded Programme on Immunization (EPI), with recommended guidelines established by the World Health Organization, is a major international effort to increase the proportion of children covered by basic immunizations against childhood diseases. Because of Africa's unusually high rates of child mortality from measles, the prevalence of tuberculosis, and in many places, substantial mortality due to neonatal tetanus, EPI plays a central role in the health strategy for Africa. In addition, the low levels of funding for health programs in Africa have forced many countries to focus their scarce resources on what are perceived as the most cost-effective interventions, which include EPI (Walsh and Warren, 1979).

In general, the vaccines that form the core of EPI programs are measles, diphtheria-pertussis-tetanus, poliomyelitis, bacille Calmette-Guérin (BCG) for tuberculosis, and tetanus for pregnant women or women of childbearing age. Each of these vaccines has been proven efficacious to varying degrees. However, vaccine efficacy does not necessarily imply that a program based on vaccinations is effective in reducing mortality. There are two reasons that programs might be less effective than suggested by the efficacy of the vaccines. First, as pointed out in Chapter 2, child mortality in Africa often results from the interaction of several diseases, frequently including malnutrition (although malnutrition, in many cases, may be a consequence of infectious and parasitic diseases). The interactions among different childhood diseases are so complex that it is difficult to estimate the effect of reducing the incidence of a single disease by using mathematical simulations. The second problem is that vaccines may be less effective in large-scale programs than in small-scale trials of their efficacy. If vaccines are stored incorrectly, used after their expiration date, not given at the appropriate age, or given to children who have already contracted a disease, the effectiveness of the immunization program can be greatly reduced. For these reasons, it is necessary to measure the actual effects of real programs.

The EPI programs in most African countries have achieved large increases in the proportion of children who receive all of the standard vaccinations. Figure 3-1 shows the proportions of children aged 12-23 months that had received all the standard vaccinations, based on data from the Demographic and Health Surveys conducted in the mid- to late 1980s. Given the relatively high levels in some countries, it is possible that these programs have had a substantial effect on infant and childhood mortality. Because most of the increase in vaccination coverage occurred after 1985, many of the children born shortly before the survey have a higher likelihood of being vaccinated than their older siblings. However, the effect of these programs on child mortality may be too recent to be evident in the available demographic data for most countries. Moreover, although the trends in immunization coverage are upward, coverage can vary greatly on

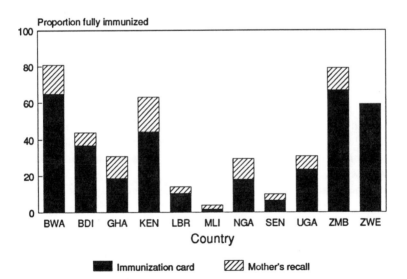

FIGURE 3-1 Proportion of fully immunized children 12-23 months of age, selected sub-Saharan African countries. NOTE: Based on immunization cards and mothers' recall. BWA—Botswana, BDI—Burundi, GHA—Ghana, KEN-Kenya, LBR—Liberia, MLI—Mali, NGA—Nigeria, SEN—Senegal, UGA—Uganda, ZMB—Zambia, ZWE—Zimbabwe. SOURCE: Demographic and Health Survey reports (see Appendix B).

a year-to-year basis, especially among programs depending on special vaccination programs.

Generally, statistics gathered for the EPI program at the national level focus on specific immunizations rather than the proportion of fully immunized children. The goal of the African Region EPI program for 1990 was to make immunizations available for all infants and to achieve coverage of at least 75 percent for all six EPI vaccines. As of August 1991, the immunization coverage for children 12 to 23 months of age in Africa was estimated to have reached 79 percent for BCG, 57 percent for the third dose of the diphtheria-pertussis-tetanus (DPT) vaccine, 56 percent for the third dose of the oral poliomyelitis vaccine, and 54 percent for the measles vaccine. Although the goals have not yet been achieved, comparison with coverage in 1982 of approximately 28 percent for BCG, 21 percent for poliomyelitis, and 18 percent for measles suggests that vaccination coverage has increased greatly as the EPI program became activated (Expanded Programme on Immunization, 1992).

The following sections examine the evidence that vaccination programs against measles, pertussis, tuberculosis, and tetanus have reduced child mortality. Most of the research on EPI programs has focused on measles. The reasons for this emphasis include the high mortality rates from measles, its relative ease of diagnosis, and the potential of program failure because of improper vaccine handling. Much less research exists on pertussis, tuberculosis in children, and tetanus. However, there are several indications of the potential effects of these programs.

We have not reviewed the literature on two of the EPI diseases: poliomyelitis and diphtheria. We have not included polio because of the low number of deaths from this disease. However, several African studies suggest that poliomyelitis vaccination campaigns can reduce the incidence of disease and paralysis (Rodrigues, 1991; Deming et al., 1992), despite the vaccine's lower efficacy in Africa than in developed countries (Oduntan, 1978; Böttinger et al., 1981; Expanded Programme on Immunization, 1990; de Swardt et al., 1990).

Diphtheria has a low incidence rate in sub-Saharan Africa because of high levels of acquired immunity, but can have a high case-fatality rate (Rodrigues, 1991). This immunity may be due to widespread, relatively mild, subclinical cases. Among children diagnosed with diphtheria, the case-fatality rate is high. Relative to other diseases, diphtheria is apparently not a major cause of death among African children. One study suggests that DPT vaccination in Sudan has reduced the incidence of diphtheria (Loevinsohn, 1990). We know very little about the role of diphtheria in African mortality because no reliable sources of community-based data exist, nor is there information about the contribution of diphtheria vaccine to the effect of vaccination programs in Africa (Rodrigues, 1991).

Several vaccines that are included in immunization programs in some parts of the African continent are not reviewed here. In particular, yellow fever and meningitis vaccines are used to control epidemics in parts of West Africa.

MEASLES

As discussed in the introduction to this chapter, measles is one of the leading causes of infant and child mortality in sub-Saharan Africa. Here, we review the state of knowledge on measles. We begin with a discussion of the epidemiology and vaccine efficacy. A discussion on why Africa may be different from other parts of the world with respect to measles follows. Measles immunization programs are then examined, with a focus on their effects, the relationship between immunization coverage and measles mortality, and program history and coverage. Finally, treatment strategies are discussed.

EPIDEMIOLOGY

Measles is caused by a paramyxovirus called morbilli. It is highly infectious and transmitted from person to person via droplet spread (sneezes or coughs) or through direct contact with nasal or throat secretions of infected persons. The incubation period of approximately 10 to 12 days is followed by cough, nasal congestion, and conjunctivitis. The characteristic rash appears about two to four days after the onset of other symptoms. The total illness generally lasts 7 to 10 days (Orenstein et al., 1986). A case of measles provides lifetime protection, and repeat cases are rare. The symptoms of the disease are well known in Africa, and there are local names for it in many languages. Common complications include otitis media (inner ear infections), laryngitis, pneumonia, diarrhea, and encephalitis.

Measles is one of the major causes of death among children in Africa. It is a contributing factor in 8 to 10 percent of deaths among African children (Ofosu-Amaah, 1983; Rodrigues, 1991). The proportion is even higher in many parts of the continent. For example, a study in Senegal in 1963-1965 found that measles deaths accounted for 26 percent of deaths among children ages 1 to 4 and 19 percent of all deaths under age 5 (Cantrelle, 1968). During epidemic years, measles can be responsible for 50 percent of all deaths at ages 1 to 4 years (Garenne and Cantrelle, 1986).

Because measles often leads to severe diarrhea or respiratory infections, it is probably an underlying cause of many more child deaths. For example, a study in Bangladesh (Clemens et al., 1988) found that measles vaccination reduced the odds of dying from diarrhea by 59 percent, the odds from respiratory illness by 22 percent, and the odds from malnutrition (i.e., "swelling or edema") by 47 percent. Feachem and Koblinsky (1983) listed measles immunization as one strategy for reducing child mortality from diarrheal diseases. They calculated that measles immunization at the age of 9-11 months, with coverage of 45 to 90 percent might avert 6-26 percent of diarrhea deaths among children less than 5 years of age.

Although respiratory and gastrointestinal infections often occur during or in the month after measles cases, excess mortality can continue for many months. Hull et al. (1983) followed children who had measles and compared their overall mortality with that of children who did not have measles. Half of the extra deaths among children who had measles occurred three to nine months after the case. Therefore, studies that ascribe death in the one to three months following a case as measles deaths may be understating the true effect of measles on mortality rates. One possible explanation for the long-term effect of measles is the growth retardation that often follows. The Kasongo Project Team (1986) documented that three months after the onset of measles, growth retardation was still apparent based on both weight-for-age and weight-for-height relative to local standards, as discussed in Chapter 5. Another possible explanation is an alteration of physical defense mechanisms or a decrease in immunocompetence because of the measles virus.

VACCINE EFFICACY

There are several measles vaccines in use today. The most common in Africa is the Schwarz vaccine, an attenuated live vaccine introduced in 1966. During the 1980s, this and other measles vaccines were modified to increase their stability and, thereby, their effectiveness. A second vaccine, the Edmonston-Zagreb, has recently been tested in high doses as a way of lowering the standard age at which the vaccination can be given.

Several studies, most of them prospective studies based in communities, have estimated the efficacy of measles vaccine, which is its ability to prevent measles when used in carefully controlled trials. In a recent clinical trial conducted in Senegal, the efficacy of the Schwarz measles vaccine given at 10 months of age was 98 percent (the 95 percent confidence interval (C.I.) was 86-100 percent; Garenne et al., 1992). A study by Hull et al. (1983) estimated that measles vaccine efficacy in The Gambia was 89 percent in children more than 9 months of age (95 percent C.I. 77-94 percent). Lamb (1988) estimated an efficacy of 90 percent for The Gambia. These estimates are close to those from Europe and North America (e.g., Miller, 1987; Rebiere et al., 1990).

However, a study by Aaby et al. (1990b) estimated a lower vaccine efficacy of only 46 percent (95 percent C.I. 7-69 percent) in Bandim district in Guinea-Bissau, among children born in 1984-1985. Even after assuming that the vaccine was not effective until 35 days after the injection, they still estimated that its efficacy was only 68 percent (95 percent C.I. 39-84 percent). This low efficacy was not due to vaccine failure since antibody tests of vaccinated children showed rates of seropositivity greater than 95 percent. It is also unlikely that this low estimate is a result of either misclassification of vaccination status or inappropriate age at vaccination.

The effectiveness of measles vaccines may be lower in field conditions than in carefully conducted studies because of inappropriate storage of the vaccine (cold chain failures), inappropriate age at vaccination, or other incorrect vaccination procedures (e.g., Cutts et al., 1990a).

A recent study of children vaccinated at the Institute of Child Health at University College Hospital in Ibadan, Nigeria (Adu et al., 1992) suggests that vaccine effectiveness might be a serious problem. Only 55 percent of children seroconverted after vaccination, and 87 percent of these had low antibody levels. The vaccines came from four different manufacturers and nine batches. The authors suggested that this low efficacy may have been a result of cold chain failures.

Attempts to measure effectiveness of large immunization programs are complicated by problems in verifying both vaccination status and measles cases. For example, a study in Mozambique found that adjustments for the estimated accuracy of mother's reports of measles cases raised the estimated vaccine efficacy from 37 to 66 percent (Cutts et al., 1990a). A similar study in Tanzania found an efficacy of 54 percent based on mother's recall of vaccination status compared to an estimate of 96 percent based on clinic cards (Killewo et al., 1991).

Garenne et al. (1992) used health cards, as well as clinical and serological records, to estimate the efficacy of vaccines delivered by the national vaccination campaigns in the study area of Niakhar, Senegal, in 1986-1987. They estimated the vaccine efficacy for those children immunized at 86 percent (95 percent C.I. 77-92 percent). This estimate represents a failure rate five times greater than that found in clinical trials using the same vaccine in the same area. Porter et al. (1990) examined vaccine efficacy in five refugee camps in Malawi. They based their calculations on the vaccination status of children who had a health card (which indicates immunizations definitely received) and estimated efficacy to be greater than 90 percent.

These studies suggest that vaccine efficacy is very high in Africa in carefully controlled studies. However, in programs, vaccine failure can be a serious problem. Therefore, we cannot simply assume that high coverage rates necessarily imply that large proportions of children are protected against measles.

There are some studies in other continents that demonstrate the effectiveness of measles vaccination in reducing mortality. For example, a study in Bangladesh (Koenig et al., 1990) found that mortality among vaccinated children ages 9 to 60 months was about 40 percent lower than among a matched group of unvaccinated children. This difference remained after controlling for differences in socioeconomic status and after several tests for selectivity in the acceptance of vaccination.[1]

WHY AFRICA MIGHT BE DIFFERENT

Measles is a more significant factor in child mortality in Africa than in other areas of the world. One reason for this higher significance is that the high fertility rates in Africa quickly replenish the population of children who have not had measles. In cities, this replenishment leads to frequent epidemics and a younger mean age of cases than was true in Europe before the availability of measles vaccine. Differences in residence patterns between Africa and other areas of the world, with extended families living in enclosed areas in some parts of Africa, can lead to higher case-fatality rates (see below).

Estimates of the case-fatality rate for measles suggest that it is unusually severe in some parts of West Africa (Aaby, 1988). The high case-fatality rate is probably not due solely to the young age distribution of cases because the epidemic in southwestern Ethiopia also exhibited very high case-fatality rates, despite 22.6 percent of cases having occurred among children aged 5 to 10 years and 5.9 percent in children 11 years or older (Lindtjorn, 1990). Although the high prevalence of malnutrition is often mentioned as a reason for high case-fatality rates, the evidence is inconclusive (see discussion of nutrition and measles in Chapter 5). It is likely that the high case-fatality rates are related to the low level of health services available in many areas and the high proportion of secondary cases in households (discussed in detail below).

Another feature of measles in Africa is that measles vaccination is effective at earlier ages than is true in developed countries because maternal antibodies wane earlier in African children. This reduction in immunity is

---

[1]The analysis conducted by Koenig et al. was based on a study carried out by Phillips et al. (1984) in which measles vaccination was offered in March 1982 to all children 9 months of age or older in two (Blocks A and C) of four intervention subareas. In November 1985, measles vaccination was expanded to the remaining two blocks (Blocks B and D). The analysis by Koenig et al. consists of all children in Blocks A and C who were immunized between 9 and 60 months during the period March 1982 to October 1985. These children were randomly matched with unvaccinated children in Blocks B and D, based on: (1) having no record of being vaccinated for measles during the study period; (2) being born in the same month and year as the corresponding matched vaccinee; and (3) the nonvaccinee having survived at least to the date of vaccination of the matched vaccinee.

apparently due to lower levels of maternal antibodies and less efficient transport of antibodies to the fetus (Black et al., 1986). There is some evidence that children born to mothers who are positive for human immunodeficiency virus (HIV) may have even poorer transport of measles antibodies and a higher risk of measles infection before age 9 months than other children (Embree et al., 1992).

The recommended age for vaccination is 9-11 months for tropical Africa, compared to 12-15 months for Europe and the United States (Kenya Ministry of Health and World Health Organization, 1977; Expanded Programme on Immunization, 1982). In some areas, programs have lowered the age for measles vaccination to 6 months. In a study in The Gambia, the efficacy dropped to 37 percent when administered at 6-8 months of age (Hull et al., 1983). Therefore, regular vaccination before 9 months of age is generally not recommended unless it is possible to provide a second dose after age 9 months. Studies of the use of high-titer vaccines (i.e., vaccines with high levels of the attenuated virus) on younger children (4-6 months) show reasonable levels of seroconversion and efficacy in preventing measles cases (Whittle et al., 1984, 1988; Aaby et al., 1988b), but low efficacy in reducing mortality (Garenne et al., 1991).

EVIDENCE OF MORTALITY AND MORBIDITY EFFECTS FROM AFRICA

There are quite a few studies of the effect of measles vaccination on both mortality and the incidence of disease in Africa. The following sections first review the evidence that vaccination against measles can reduce mortality in Africa, then the evidence that programs have reduced the incidence of measles cases.

There are several studies that examine the effect of measles vaccination on child mortality rates in sub-Saharan Africa. These studies can be divided into two groups: (1) studies that measure the effect of regular measles immunization programs on mortality, and (2) studies of effects in model programs limited to special research areas. The former evaluations are closer to our main interest because they examine the effect of large-scale programs. The second group of studies demonstrates what can be accomplished in carefully managed programs. These studies provide evidence of the relationship between changes in the incidence of measles and reductions in overall child mortality.

Effects of General Measles Immunization Programs

Garenne et al. (1985) studied the effect of the national vaccination program in Senegal. The program increased coverage with measles vaccine nationally from a few percent in the early 1960s to 74 percent for 1967 and 1968. After 1968, coverage dropped for several years. Garenne et al. (1985) provided data showing that the annual number of measles cases reported nationally dropped by 35 percent in 1967-1971 compared to 1963-1966, corresponding to the national vaccination campaign in 1967-1969. They also show that the proportion of deaths ascribed to measles decreased substantially in the two rural study areas of Ngayokhème and Ndemène (among deaths at ages 0-14 years) and in Dakar (deaths at all ages).

After a brief drop, vaccination coverage in Senegal remained greater than about 75 percent nationally for 1974-1979 (Garenne et al., 1985). Even so, the number of children seeking medical attention for measles returned to high levels. In addition, the proportion of child deaths due to measles returned to high levels for 1972-1978 in Ngayokhème and Ndemène, areas covered by continuous registration of deaths.

Two studies in Guinea-Bissau, one in an urban area (Bandim; Aaby et al., 1984b) and one in a rural area (Quinhamel; Aaby et al., 1984a), were natural experiments brought about by the introduction of measles vaccination in preexisting research areas. In Bandim, the mortality rate among children aged 6-35 months was 127 deaths per 1,000 in 1979. After a measles vaccination campaign, the rate dropped to 47 in 1980 and 48 in 1981. During 1980 and 1981, the mortality rates for vaccinated children were much lower than the rates among unvaccinated children (Aaby et al., 1984b). Mortality was also lower among vaccinated children than among children who had previously had measles. In Quinhamel, the rates were 107 per 1,000 in 1979 and 98 per 1,000 in 1980. After a measles vaccination campaign in early 1981, the rate was 44 among the vaccinated and 72 among the unvaccinated (Aaby et al., 1984a). Quinhamel was the only one of five rural areas studied where measles was a problem during the study period (Aaby, 1988).

Effects of Measles Vaccination
in Field Trials and Model Programs

There have been several field trials in defined study populations that were specifically designed to measure the effects of vaccination on mortality. In addition, several model programs have demonstrated the potential of programs. These studies offer more information than vaccine trials because they provide estimates of both the direct and the indirect effects of vaccination. In particular, the measured effects from these studies include the reduction of mortality from diarrhea, respiratory infections, and malnutrition. In vaccine trials, some of these deaths would not be recognized as resulting from measles. If continued for a sufficiently long time, these studies also can show changes in the frequency of epidemics and the resulting change in the age distribution of cases. Similarly, these studies are often superior to evaluations of general health programs since they are often based on more scientific study designs. For example, they can include control areas, randomization, or estimation of the effect of the program on those who actually received services.

However, these special studies can present a misleading picture of the likely effect of real programs. One reason is that large-scale programs rarely match the high level of supervision and training achieved in smaller programs. It is possible, therefore, that large-scale programs might have more cold chain failures and be less likely to reach the most vulnerable parts of the population. A second reason is that it is easier to carry out field trials in populations where measles is a frequent health problem. In particular, it is not feasible to test the effect of a measles program in an area that experiences measles epidemics only every three to five years. It is also more difficult to carry out these studies in urban areas because of high rates of population mobility. Finally, areas used in research studies often have better access to general health services than other rural areas.

Vaccine Field Trial in Khombole, Senegal

Garenne and Cantrelle (1986) estimated the efficacy of the Schwarz vaccine using data from field trials in Khombole, Senegal, in 1965-1968. They found that the proportion dying between ages 6 months and 10 years was 26 percent lower among children in the area receiving vaccinations than among children in the control area. It is possible that these results might be affected by other factors related to the selection of the children who were vaccinated. Vaccinations were offered to all children in the vaccination zone. Sixty percent of eligible children were vaccinated in 1965 and 86 percent were vaccinated in 1967. However, because of the nature of the program and the lack of large socioeconomic differentials within the study population, it is unlikely that the results are an artifact of selectivity.

Kasongo Project in Zaire

The Kasongo Project Team (1981) compared mortality in two areas of rural Zaire. In one area, a measles vaccination program achieved a coverage rate of 83 percent among the cohort born between September 1974 and October 1975.[2] In the test area, the mortality rate between 7 and 35 months

---

[2]Measles vaccination was offered to 306 children, of whom 83 percent accepted and were vaccinated. However, the proportion of child-months of observation that were protected by

of age was 95 deaths per 1,000 for the unvaccinated cohort born between June 1973 and August 1974. The rate dropped to 48 per 1,000 for the cohort covered by the vaccination program. In the control area, the rate fell from 80 to 69 over the same period. Therefore, mortality was reduced by 36 deaths per 1,000 more in the vaccination area than in the control area, a difference that was not statistically significant. The Kasongo Project Team suggested that the gains from vaccination appeared to have been reversed at later ages. This conclusion is not warranted by the data they present. Mortality at ages 22-35 months of age increased by 7 per 1,000 in the control area but by only 1 per 1,000 in the vaccination area. These estimates were not significantly different. Data for children beyond age 36 months are not presented.

Pahou Primary Health Care Project, Benin

The Pahou project measured the effect of primary health care services established in 16 villages 30 kilometers from Cotonou, Benin. Velema et al. (1991) matched each child who died between 4 and 35 months of age with up to four controls of the same age and sex from the same village. A comparison of the vaccination status of cases and controls showed that children vaccinated before 12 months of age experienced a relative risk of death between 4 and 35 months of 0.36, compared to nonvaccinated children (95 percent C.I. 0.16-0.81 times).[3] However, vaccination after 12 months of age was not associated with reduced mortality (relative risk: 1.02 times, 95 percent C.I. 0.43-2.41 times). These results remained after the addition of controls for socioeconomic status, nutritional status, and other measures of the effect of primary health care. These data cannot be used to estimate the change in mortality associated with vaccination because the study did not provide mortality rates for the population.[4]

Estimates of Effect from Cases of Vaccine Failure

A study in Guinea-Bissau by Aaby et al. (1989) compared children who seroconverted after measles vaccination with a group for whom the vaccina-

---

immunization was much lower. The estimated coverage was only 58 percent based on a comparison of the person-months of observation for the program area (their group 1) and for the vaccinated children in the program area (group 1v).

[3]Vaccinations in control children after the age at death of the cases were not included in the analysis.

[4]The "overall mortality rate" quoted in the article is not a true population mortality rate since it is based only on cases and controls. This rate is therefore an artifact of the number of controls (surviving children) chosen per case (deceased children).

tion failed. The proportion dying between ages 6 and 35 months from all causes was less than one-third the rate among those who seroconverted (4.5 per 1,000 compared to 15.1 per 1,000). The advantage of this study is that the unprotected children were selected by the random timing of vaccine failure. Therefore, there is no reason to believe that the unvaccinated children in the study differed from the vaccinated children in socioeconomic status, maternal beliefs, or any other potentially confounding characteristic.

Effect of Programs on Incidence in Africa

Studies of the mortality effect of measles immunization demonstrate the effectiveness of programs based on the standard vaccination regimen. If these programs based on the standard vaccines and standard age schedule for vaccination are having an effect, we should be able to determine their effectiveness through changes in the incidence of measles or the incidence of cases treated at health facilities. If a large enough number of children at risk of measles receive a potent vaccine to reduce the incidence of disease, it should be possible to document the effect on disease incidence.

Changes in the observed incidence of measles can be compared with the predictions of mathematical models. These models predict two changes that may occur when vaccination coverage increases. First, there might be a change in the frequency of measles epidemics. It is not easy to predict the change that will result from a given level of coverage because populations differ substantially in the degrees of contact between children. However, if vaccination coverage increases sufficiently, epidemics will be less frequent during the years immediately after the start of the vaccination program (Cutts et al., 1991). Second, there might be a substantial change in the age distribution of cases, which is discussed later in the chapter.

Several studies have documented dramatic changes in the incidence of measles following large increases in vaccination coverage. One of the earliest demonstrations of the potential effect of measles vaccination in Africa is based on data from 10 countries in West Africa that were included in a regional program to eradicate smallpox and control measles that began in 1967. By aggregating the data from about 150 geographical units in these countries according to the start of the vaccination program, Foege (1971) showed that the number of measles cases dropped by 54 percent in the year following, compared to the 12 months preceding, the start of the program.

Foege (1971) also presented more detailed data from The Gambia that provide a dramatic demonstration of the reduction of measles cases after the first national measles vaccination campaign. Figure 3-2 shows the number of measles cases in five regions of The Gambia during each four-week period of 1967 and 1968. Each region had a measles campaign during

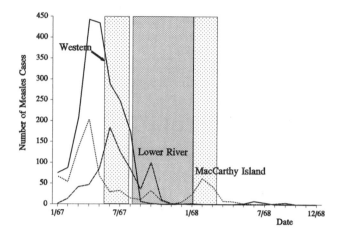

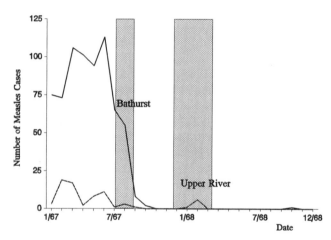

FIGURE 3-2 Effect of measles vaccination coverage on measles cases (by four-week period), five areas of The Gambia. NOTE: Shaded areas indicate periods of inital vaccination campaign in each area. SOURCE: Foege (1971).

different months of 1967 and early 1968. The campaign targeted all children aged 6 months to 4 years and achieved a coverage rate of 96 percent. Although the numbers of measles cases had begun to drop in several of the regions, they dropped dramatically, to zero in many cases, following the campaign in each region. By June 1968, measles transmission had been interrupted. There were only 16 cases during 1969 and 1970, and most of them were imported.

The campaigns begun in the late 1960s did not lead to a large-scale program of continuous vaccination with high coverage rates. However, data are available for several countries that increased their vaccination coverage rates during the 1980s. For example, vaccination coverage in Malawi increased from 10 percent in 1976-1978 to about 60 percent in 1985-1987. Surveillance data show that the number of cases in the later period was only about half of the number reported a decade earlier (Expanded Programme on Immunization, 1989). Similarly, Cutts et al. (1991) found that the reported number of cases of measles in Burundi decreased by more than 50 percent between 1981 and 1988. Vaccination coverage in 1986-1988 averaged more than 60 percent, compared to about 20 percent in 1980. They also found that in Rwanda, the reported incidence in 1988, when coverage was greater than 80 percent, was only 3 percent of the rate reported before the start of immunization program. Similarly, data for Lesotho show a large drop in reported incidence rates as vaccination coverage increased.

Dabis et al. (1988) examined the decline in reported measles cases in Pointe-Noire, Congo, during implementation of the Expanded Programme on Immunization, which began there in January 1982. The estimated coverage rate increased to 31 and 37 percent, respectively, in 1982 and 1983, and to 47 percent in 1984 and 1985. A community survey in 1985 estimated that 54 percent of the children 12-23 months of age had documented evidence of vaccination against measles. Measles had been endemic in Pointe-Noire since at least 1979, with annual epidemics. Data on hospital admissions for measles showed that the monthly number of measles cases dropped to very low figures during late 1983 and early 1984, instead of rising for the annual epidemic. In addition, between 1983 and 1985 (both epidemic years), the hospitalization rate for measles among children 9 to 23 months of age dropped by 49 percent. This decline was associated with an increase in the proportion of hospitalized cases less than 9 months of age from 13 to 17 percent.

A study in Yaoundé, Cameroon, in 1974-1979 showed that the number of recorded measles cases dropped by 44 percent when the cold chain was improved and the minimum age at vaccination was increased from 6 to 9 months (Heymann et al., 1983). Despite the increase in the minimum age at vaccination, the number of cases dropped in all age groups, including less than 9 months.

NONLINEARITIES IN RELATIONSHIP BETWEEN COVERAGE AND EFFECT

The potential effect of measles vaccination on mortality can vary substantially across populations and programs. First, the potential effect of programs will differ according to the epidemiology of measles in various populations, including features such as the frequency of epidemics and the intensity of infections. Second, the relationship between vaccination coverage and mortality is not simple. For example, a 40 percent coverage rate might be sufficient to disrupt a pattern of annual epidemics in a small town with low fertility rates. A large city with high fertility would require a much higher coverage rate to achieve the same result. The studies reviewed above demonstrate that a vaccination program in Africa that reduces the incidence of the disease will reduce mortality as well. However, it is difficult to estimate how much mortality will decline in any given situation.

The following sections describe the factors that determine the relationship between vaccine coverage and mortality reduction.

Vaccination and Frequency of Epidemics

An increase in the proportion of the population protected by vaccination can change the whole epidemiology of the disease. For example, an effective vaccination campaign can virtually stop transmission of the disease for two to three years. The level of coverage required to achieve this result depends on the density of the population, the fertility rate, and local practices that affect transmission rates (e.g., migration patterns).

Effect of Vaccination on Age Distribution of Cases

The age distribution of cases is important for two reasons. First, because case-fatality rates are highest among cases under 12 months of age, a change in the age distribution of cases can change the case-fatality rate. Second, in some populations, the best evidence of the effect of the program comes from a change in the number and age distribution of cases seen at hospitals and health centers.

Programs designed to increase the coverage of measles vaccination generally reduce incidence rates at all ages. However, because the biggest declines are often concentrated at ages 12-35 months, there is often a change in the age distribution of cases observed in hospitals and clinics. A sudden increase in program effort often leads to a temporary drop in the proportion of cases at 12-35 months of age and an increase in the proportion of cases among children more than 5 years of age. The proportion over age 5 increases in some populations because without vaccination, most children get measles before this age. If vaccination coverage increases the interval between epidemics or leads to smaller isolated epidemics, some children escape measles until later ages. For example, Aaby et al. (1988a) reported that in Guinea-Bissau, greater vaccination coverage increased the proportion of cases over age 5 from 22 to 29 percent. Change in the age distribution of cases is a useful indicator of program effectiveness. These changes can often be documented through surveillance systems when complete population surveys are not available. For example, in the city of Maputo, Mozambique,

TABLE 3-1 Proportion of Measles Cases Among
Children Over Age 5 Years in Areas Where
Vaccination Coverage Has Remained High

Country	Vaccine Coverage (%)	Reported Cases ≥5 years (%)
Burundi	57	35
Lesotho	78	62
Rwanda	86	31
Swaziland	74	41
The Gambia	90	50

SOURCES: National data from Cutts et al. (1991), except for The
Gambia, for which data are from Keneba, reported by Lamb (1988).

vaccination coverage increased from 42 percent in 1982 to 86 percent in
1986. Data on cases reported by health centers showed a shift in the proportion of cases over 5 years of age from about 10 percent in 1982-1983 to
28 percent in 1986 and 40 percent in 1987 (Cutts et al., 1990b).

After a program has maintained high coverage levels for several years,
the proportion of children over age 5 protected by vaccination will increase.
However, that proportion can still remain high. Table 3-1 presents the
proportion of cases over age 5 in five areas in which vaccination coverage
had remained greater than 50 percent for several years. After vaccination
levels have remained high for many years, it may be useful to consider
providing a second dose to older children. This strategy will protect those
who were missed initially and those who were not protected adequately by
the first dose, although the mortality effect will be lower with the second
dose than with the first.

Increases in vaccination coverage may result in an increase in the proportion of cases less than 12 months of age. Because the case-fatality rate
is highest among infants, increasing the proportion of cases in this age
group is likely to raise the overall case-fatality rate. During the years when
coverage is high, there are fewer cases among children age 1-3 because of
the vaccination, and still fewer cases over age 5 because these children have
either been vaccinated or had measles. Therefore, the proportion of cases
under 1 year of age is likely to increase, at least in the short run. For
example, in Pointe-Noire, Congo, the proportion of hospitalized cases at 0-8
months of age increased from 13 to 17 percent when vaccination coverage
increased from about 30-35 percent to 45 percent (Dabis et al., 1988). Similarly,
Taylor et al. (1988) reported on the trends in measles in Kinshasa, Zaire.
Between 1977 and 1983, coverage with measles vaccine increased from 37
to 62 percent among children age 12-23 months. Between 1983 and 1985 it

remained between about 50 and 60 percent. Despite this high rate of coverage, measles epidemics continued in alternate years between 1980 and 1985. Surveillance data from hospitals and health centers and a community survey showed that the proportion of cases among children less than 1 year of age increased with increasing vaccination coverage.

The new equilibrium age distribution of cases depends on the pattern of measles in the population and the nature of the vaccination program. For example, in Maputo, Mozambique, the proportion of reported cases less than 9 months of age increased slightly from 19 percent in 1982 to 22 percent in 1985. The proportion then dropped to 15 percent in 1987 (Cutts et al., 1990b). On the other hand, Aaby et al. (1988a) report almost no change in Guinea-Bissau in the proportion of cases under age 12 months— rising only from 17 to 18 percent.

Data from health facilities can exaggerate the increase in the proportion of cases among infants. Since younger children often have more severe cases (in part because they are more likely to be secondary cases), infants are overrepresented at health facilities. Because vaccination reduces the number of cases at 12-18 months of age (which also have higher severity), the proportion of hospitalized patients under 1 year is apt to increase substantially. In Machakos, Kenya, the percentage of cases among infants was twice as large for hospitalized cases as for all cases (Muller et al., 1977). In Kinshasa, 45 percent of cases reported in hospitals and clinics between 1980 and 1985 were less than 1 year of age, while in a community study, only 37 percent were infants (Taylor et al., 1988). Similarly, in an outbreak in Kampala, Uganda, in 1990, 28 percent of measles patients in hospitals were less than 9 months of age. However, a community survey about three months later reported that only 11 percent of cases were children under 12 months of age (Expanded Programme on Immunization, 1991).

It is important to stress that these changes in the age distribution of cases do not reflect changes in the incidence rate among infants. Vaccination programs reduce the incidence of measles among children under age 12 months. However, the case rates at older ages often decline more than those at the youngest ages, and therefore the proportion of cases at each age will change.

As coverage increases, the proportion of cases associated with vaccine failure will increase. This shift does not imply an increase in the proportion of vaccinations that fail. Instead, it reflects the increasing number who are vaccinated and consequently at risk of vaccine failure. Therefore, it is not possible to monitor changes in program effectiveness merely by documenting the number of vaccine failures or the proportion of cases associated with vaccine failure.

Changes in the Proportion of Secondary Cases

One reason case-fatality rates decrease with age is that younger children are more likely to become infected through contact with an older household member. Numerous studies have demonstrated that secondary cases of measles in a household (i.e., those who are infected by another household member) have a higher case-fatality rate than isolated cases (Aaby et al., 1984a,c; Hull, 1988; Koster, 1988; Lamb, 1988; Pison and Bonneuil, 1988; Aaby and Leeuwenberg, 1990; Garenne and Aaby, 1990). The higher case fatality may be a result of higher doses of virus associated with closer continuous contact between children in the same household.

If a vaccination program reduces the proportion of secondary cases, the case-fatality rate can drop substantially. For example, Aaby et al. (1988a) reported that the proportion of isolated cases increased from 16 percent before the vaccination program to 33 percent over the next three years. This change was largely responsible for a drop in the case-fatality rate of children under age 12 months from 28 to 17 percent—although this latter figure is still very high.

The change in the proportion of secondary cases will depend on the way in which vaccinations are distributed in the population. For example, if vaccination coverage remains low in a segment of the population with large families (e.g., polygamous households), then the proportion of secondary cases could increase. On the other hand, as the interval between epidemics increases, a larger proportion of cases will be children over age 5 who are apt to have one or more younger siblings. During an outbreak in a primary school in Burundi, 25 of the 28 cases were primary cases in their household. These led to 31 secondary cases, 90 percent of which were younger siblings (Cutts et al., 1991).

When vaccination coverage increases enough to delay measles epidemics for several years, small epidemics can arise from cases that originate at a health facility (e.g., Expanded Programme on Immunization, 1986; Chahnazarian et al., 1993). Such outbreaks occur because the health facilities bring together a number of children at risk of measles. A case-control study in a child health clinic on the outskirts of Abidjan, Côte d'Ivoire, during a measles epidemic showed that attending the clinic was associated with a 30 percent additional risk (95 percent C.I. 9-102 percent) of contracting measles (Expanded Programme on Immunization, 1986). In this population, where coverage of measles vaccination was 64 percent, about 67 percent of cases were attributable to attendance at the clinic during the epidemic.

A study of measles cases in Mbeya, Tanzania (Burgess et al., 1986), suggested that these "nosocomial" cases may have a higher case-fatality rate. These data provide a strong argument for vaccinating all unvaccinated children who attend any child health clinic, including those with fever and rashes that are often incorrectly assumed to be contraindications for vaccination.

Other Factors

Other factors can influence the effect of programs. First, there is a report that cases of measles among vaccinated children (e.g., vaccine failures) have a lower case-fatality rate than those among unvaccinated children (Aaby et al., 1986). However, another study failed to demonstrate this difference (Lamb, 1988). Second, Aaby and his colleagues have demonstrated that in Guinea-Bissau, children exposed to measles before 6 months of age have higher mortality than other children (Aaby et al., 1990a, 1993), even though about 75 percent of both the exposed and the unexposed were later vaccinated against measles. This difference does not appear to be due to selectivity factors determining who gets vaccinated or to socioeconomic differentials. The effect of exposure to measles appears to last for 2 to 3 years following exposure. Therefore, it is possible that vaccination programs might reduce mortality by reducing exposure to measles before age 6 months in addition to the direct effect of vaccination at a later age.

PROGRAM HISTORY, COVERAGE, AND QUALITY

In 1966, mass vaccination campaigns were begun in West and Central Africa through a 20-country program for smallpox eradication and measles control (Ofosu-Amaah, 1983). Consequently, vaccine coverage increased significantly in the late 1960s and early 1970s. Although these programs were successful in vaccinating large numbers of children, there were also many technical and managerial problems. Coverage rates dropped as these problems became apparent and program efforts slackened. After the World Health Assembly in 1974, the World Health Organization launched the Expanded Programme on Immunization. In 1978, the World Conference on Primary Health Care held in Alma-Ata identified immunization as an essential element of primary care. These renewed efforts were based on the newer, more heat-stable measles vaccines and a major programmatic emphasis on technical training of local personnel.

The most current estimates (early 1990s) for sub-Saharan African countries suggest a measles vaccination coverage rate of about 52 percent. These figures compare favorably with 1981 estimates of about 30 to 33 percent (International Science and Technology Institute, 1990; United Nations Children's Fund, 1991; Expanded Programme on Immunization, 1992; Nigerian Federal Office of Statistics and Institute for Resource Development, 1992). Figure 3-3 illustrates the changes in coverage rates at the national level between the early 1980s and early 1990s. These estimates are very rough;

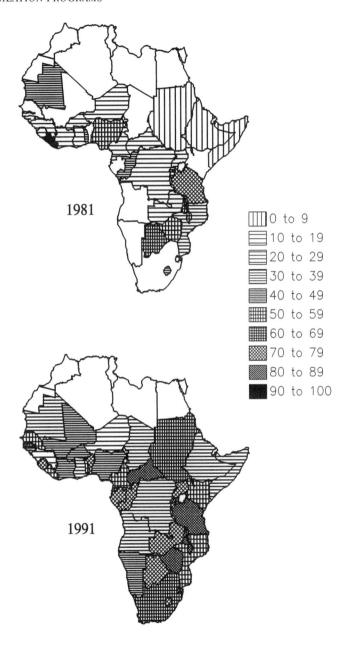

FIGURE 3-3 Proportions of children aged 12-23 months who have received measles vaccination, countries of sub-Saharan Africa, 1981 and 1991. SOURCES: 1981 data from United Nations Children's Fund (1991); 1991 data from International Science and Technology Institute (1990) and Expanded Programme on Immunization (1992).

many are based on administrative records rather than population surveys. Even the data based on surveys generally have a 95 percent confidence interval of at least ±10 percent. Surveys generally accept only vaccination cards, which provide information on when specific vaccinations were given— rather than relying on mothers' recall—as proof of vaccination. Estimated coverage may be biased downward if women lose or do not have vaccination cards to show to the interviewer or if programs run short of cards. On the other hand, accepting a mother's recall of past vaccinations might bias the estimate upward.

Gareaballah and Loevinsohn (1989) tested the accuracy of mother's recall of measles vaccinations in the Sudan. They interviewed illiterate mothers who had vaccination cards. They found that 87 percent of mothers whose child had been vaccinated reported correctly (the sensitivity) as did 79 percent of mothers whose child had not been vaccinated (the specificity). Therefore, they conclude that in the Sudan, limiting estimates of vaccination coverage to card-verified cases would lead to an underestimation of coverage. The coverage rate based on cards was only 43 percent compared to 66 percent based on cards and mothers' reports.

Moreover, coverage can vary substantially from year to year, especially in countries that rely on periodic national campaign days and those plagued by political problems. If coverage surveys are often carried out to demonstrate program success, these surveys may give more emphasis to high-coverage years. Because the estimates for 1981 are more likely to be based on administrative records, and coverage rates were changing rapidly at that time, estimates for 1981 are probably less reliable than those for 1991.

Despite the data problems, we can safely conclude that many more African children are currently protected by measles vaccination than were 10 years ago. The countries that have the lowest coverage rates are often those that have been affected by other economic and political problems (e.g., Ethiopia, Somalia, and Angola). Other countries may have experienced declines in coverage because of political problems since these estimates were made (e.g., Liberia and Zaire).

In places with relatively high coverage, it is possible that a small additional percentage in vaccination coverage can have an important effect on mortality. First, vaccination coverage is generally higher among children living in urban areas (where health facilities are often concentrated) and among children whose mothers are educated (Boerma et al., 1990). Mothers' education is not just a reflection of urban status. For example, a study in two periurban towns in The Gambia demonstrated significant differences between the educational status of both the mothers and the fathers of vaccinated and unvaccinated children within a single urban area (Hanlon et al., 1988). Expanding vaccination coverage in rural areas and among children with uneducated parents might have a greater effect than providing vaccinations to the more advantaged parts of the population. Second, at higher levels of coverage, changes in the frequency of epidemics might provide the best protection for children under the recommended age for vaccination.

TREATMENT OF MEASLES (INCLUDING VITAMIN A)

The thrust of current programs is to reduce measles through vaccination, but there are still a large number of measles cases each year. The case-fatality rate among hospitalized cases of measles is often 10 to 15 percent (Kimati and Lyaruu, 1976; Dabis et al., 1988; Fischer, 1988). One strategy for combating measles cases is through improved treatment of complications, such as diarrhea and acute respiratory infections. Reduction in these illnesses can reduce measles-related mortality. (See Chapter 4 for discussions of case management of diarrheal diseases and ARI.) Moreover, recent research has suggested that treatment with vitamin A may reduce case fatality in hospitalized patients, as discussed in more detail in Chapter 5. Because in much of Africa, many children with severe cases of measles receive treatment in a hospital or health center, vitamin A treatment has the potential to have a substantial effect on case fatality.

A study of children hospitalized with measles in Kinshasa showed that among children less than 2 years of age, low serum vitamin A levels are associated with increased risk of dying (Markowitz et al., 1989). After controlling for muscle wasting, low white blood cell levels, and pneumonia at admission, those with vitamin A stores of less than 5 micrograms per deciliter had a case-fatality rate 2.9 times (95 percent C.I. 1.3-6.8) greater than those with higher serum levels. Among children 24-60 months of age, serum vitamin A was not significantly associated with increased risk of death (relative risk 1.2; 95 percent C.I. 0.2-7.8). This study demonstrated a relationship between measles and serum vitamin A levels, but it did not prove that depletion of vitamin A levels is part of the causal chain leading to death. However, reduced vitamin A levels probably increase the risk of pneumonia and diarrhea.

The first trial of the efficacy of vitamin A in the treatment of measles was carried out by Barclay et al. (1987) in Tanzania. This study showed lower mortality among measles cases under age 2 who received vitamin A (probability less than .05), but no difference among cases over age 2. For all ages, the difference between the treatment and comparison groups was not significant (probability of .13). A trial in Cape Town, South Africa (Hussey and Klein, 1990) also showed significantly lower mortality among measles cases treated with vitamin A (relative risk 0.21 times; 95 percent C.I. 0.05-0.94).

Coutsoudis et al. (1991) ran a randomized trial in Durban, South Africa, limited to cases of measles in African children under 2 years of age who presented with both pneumonia and diarrhea complications. Only one death occurred—to a child receiving the placebo. However, there was a significant difference over a seven-day follow-up in the duration of pneumonia, with the vitamin A group having a mean duration of 3.8 days compared to 5.7 for the controls (probability less than .05). There were similar differences between the durations of diarrhea and fever, although these were not statistically significant. Of the vitamin A-treated children, 96 percent recovered fully within seven days, compared to only 65 percent among controls (probability less than .0002). Although the supplemented children showed better recovery in the seven-day follow-up, measles mortality can continue for many months after the infection because of its debilitating consequences.

SUMMARY

Several studies demonstrate that measles vaccination programs can greatly increase child survival in Africa. This conclusion is strengthened by the wide variety of research designs employed in these studies. These range from case control (Velema et al., 1991), to comparisons of vaccine failures with other children (Aaby et al., 1989), to comparison of program and nonprogram areas (Kasongo Project Team, 1981). The variety of research designs makes it difficult to compare the exact magnitude of the effect of programs in different settings. However, this variety increases our confidence in the overall conclusion.

Although measles vaccination is estimated to have a large effect on child mortality, we must note that these studies cover only a small part of the continent. The studies in Senegal, The Gambia, and Guinea-Bissau were all carried out in coastal zones in areas very close to each other. The study in Benin was also carried out in a coastal area of West Africa. Only the Kasongo project in Zaire was in a noncoastal area outside West Africa. Therefore, it is risky to extrapolate from these studies to estimate the number of deaths prevented by measles vaccination in other parts of the region.

In addition, in some of the areas where the effectiveness of measles vaccination has been demonstrated, there is evidence that the efficacy may have been quite low at other times. For example, the studies by Aaby and his colleagues demonstrated that the measles vaccination program in Bandim, Guinea-Bissau, reduced child mortality during 1979-1981 (Aaby et al., 1984b). However, a later study showed that vaccine efficacy was no more than 68 percent in Bandim among children born in 1984-1985 (Aaby et al., 1990b).

Similarly, Garenne et al. (1985) showed that in Senegal the number of reported measles cases and the proportion of mortality attributed to measles dropped in several areas after the national vaccination campaign in 1966-1968. However, both reported cases and measles mortality returned to high levels during 1972-1978. Garenne et al. (1992) also examined vaccine efficacy during the national vaccination campaign in one rural area in 1986-1987. Vaccine efficacy was reasonable (86 percent), but below the levels achieved in clinical trials in the same area.

These studies suggest that even in areas where measles vaccination has been demonstrated to be very effective in reducing mortality, the health programs did not always maintain high levels of effectiveness. This lack of effectiveness is supported by occasional reports of high failure rates in other programs (e.g., Cutts et al., 1990a; Adu et al., 1992). The evidence from some areas suggests that large-scale programs can succeed in reducing the incidence of measles (e.g., Foege, 1971; Dabis et al., 1988; Expanded Programme on Immunization, 1989; Cutts et al., 1991; Kambarami et al., 1991). However, program vigilance in necessary to ensure a reasonable level of vaccine efficacy in routine programs.

Measles vaccination programs are not likely to eliminate measles from Africa in the near future. Therefore, there will continue to be cases of measles that require treatment, especially among children who are too young to be vaccinated according to the standard vaccination schedule. These younger children have higher risks of measles mortality in addition to elevated risks from the diarrhea, pneumonia, and malnutrition that frequently accompany measles.

Studies suggest that vitamin A supplementation may reduce measles mortality. However, evaluation of treatment strategies for measles cases continues to be a pressing need. Studies need to be conducted that include longer follow-up of cases and controls to ensure that increases in survival to hospital discharge represent long-term gains and not just short-term abatement of the underlying risks.

PERTUSSIS (WHOOPING COUGH)

Although a commonly occurring and often debilitating disease, whooping cough has been a neglected subject of research throughout the world and in developing countries in particular. Mortimer (1988) notes that in preindustrial Britain, the lack of earlier recorded history of pertussis may have been due to the preoccupation of physicians with other severe infections, such as plague, typhus, and smallpox, leaving the care of pertussis to mothers and other caregivers. The case would appear to be the same in contemporary Africa. A recent editorial in the *South African Medical Journal* (1989) noted a visible lack of interest in this important disease by researchers and physicians alike.

One possible explanation for this persistent lack of attention is that pertussis is a less visible infectious disease than others. It is characterized primarily by a cough, a symptom that can be caused by many other organisms. Although a frequent cause of death, whooping cough rarely kills in a quick dramatic way, as measles, smallpox, and cholera do. Pertussis is also more difficult to document both bacteriologically and serologically than many other diseases.

PERTUSSIS IN DEVELOPED COUNTRIES

Epidemiology

Whooping cough is a bacterial respiratory infection caused by *Bordetella pertussis*. *Bordetella parapertussis*, a closely related organism, can produce a similar disease, although its incidence seems to be 20 times lower than *B. pertussis* (Muller and Leeuwenburg, 1985). Cases of pertussis-like diseases have also been attributed to *B. bronchiseptica* and to different viruses. The incubation period is generally considered to be 9 or 10 days. During the first week, the symptoms are mild (cough, fever). The cough later becomes spasmodic and is often followed by a characteristic whoop, bluish coloring of the skin, and vomiting. This phase can last several weeks. Recovery is slow and gradual, and the cough may persist for many weeks (Mortimer, 1988).

The classical clinical picture of severe cases among older children is usually easily recognized by medical personnel and even by parents themselves. However, infants often have atypical symptoms, and mild forms of the disease are seen at all ages, especially in isolated cases outside major epidemics, and among vaccinated children. Culture of *B. pertussis* in the laboratory is also difficult. Even with laboratory confirmation, the algorithms for diagnosis have relatively low sensitivities and specificities (Mortimer, 1988; Patriarca et al., 1988). For example, Patriarca et al. (1988) studied four different serologic tests for diagnosing cases of pertussis. By combining the presence of cough for at least two weeks with each of these tests individually, they achieved specificities ranging from 75 to 90 percent with sensitivities ranging from 82 to 91 percent. Without the serology, they could only achieve a specificity of 80 percent with a sensitivity of 50 percent or less.

Whooping cough is a relatively frequent cause of death in developing countries. Sudden death from asphyxia due to obstruction of the airway may occur in the most severe cases. Furthermore, *B. pertussis* infection may induce pulmonary, encephalitic, and nutritional complications. Pulmonary changes may be caused by *B. pertussis* itself or, more frequently, by secondary invasion of other microorganisms such as streptococci or pneumococci. These changes may be sufficiently severe to compromise respiratory function and cause death. Acute encephalopathy may cause convulsions, altered consciousness, permanent brain damage, or death. The persistent vomiting after the cough can also induce severe malnutrition, dehydration, and later death (Morley, 1966; Mata, 1978). In addition, pertussis may aggravate other infectious diseases such as measles and tuberculosis.

Whooping cough is transmitted from person to person by droplet spread (e.g., during coughing or sneezing) and usually occurs in epidemics. Virtually all children are susceptible to whooping cough from birth. Most children are infected before age 15 years, and in unvaccinated populations, the incidence, periodicity, and dynamics of whooping cough epidemics are similar to measles epidemics. A case generally confers lifetime immunity.

Pertussis is highly contagious after infection and the onset of cold-like symptoms, which occur one to two weeks before the typical whooping cough begins. Mortality from pertussis can be controlled by proper case management based on antibiotic therapy. The cough may last for one to two months in cases not treated with antibiotics (typically erythromycin, which is an expensive drug in Africa). In the untreated case, the person may remain communicable for 4-5 weeks. Among those receiving treatment, the period of infectiousness usually lasts only 5-7 days after beginning therapy (Benenson, 1985).

Vaccine Efficacy

The main strategy for reducing pertussis mortality is immunization programs. A first generation of killed whole-cell vaccines was developed before World War II, but gave poor results. A second generation of whole-cell vaccines combined with other antigens was marketed around 1950. The diphtheria-pertussis-tetanus vaccine is a major component of national immunization programs. However, the pertussis vaccine has not only a relatively low efficacy but also infrequent side effects, such as convulsions, high fevers, and brain dysfunction, and has been the object of major controversies (Miller et al., 1982; Feery, 1984; Hinman, 1984; Hinman and Koplan, 1984). It is still not recommended in some European countries. A third generation of vaccines, the so-called acellular vaccines, has been developed and used in Japan for many years. Several other formulas are under study.

The protective efficacy of the vaccine depends very much on the definition of a case. The vaccine seems to have virtually no capacity to protect against the infection, defined as the presence of the pathogen and at least one day of cough. However, it seems to protect against the severe forms of disease, and probably against death. Studies in the United States and in the United Kingdom have shown that vaccination reduces the severity of the disease, measured by duration of symptoms, mean number of coughing spasms, number of complications, and admission to hospital (Cherry, 1984; Pollock et al., 1984).

One dose of the vaccine provides little protection, and three to four injections are needed to provide maximum protection. In an outbreak investigation in Atlanta (Broome et al., 1981), the efficacy of three injections of whole-cell pertussis vaccine was estimated at 94 percent (95 percent C.I. 75-99 percent). Another smaller study in Maryland reported by Cherry (1984) found an efficacy of 89 percent among children aged 0-9 years. In England and Wales, protective efficacy was estimated in 10 different studies; results varied from 31 to 87 percent, with a mean of 57 percent (Cherry, 1984). The largest and most comprehensive study conducted in England and Wales (Fine and Clarkson, 1984) estimated the efficacy at 56 percent (95 percent C.I. 50-61 percent).

The World Health Organization currently recommends that children in developing countries receive three injections of DPT at intervals of at least four weeks. The first injection should be given as soon as possible after 6 weeks of age. In many countries, children are rarely fully vaccinated before age 6 months, creating a high-risk period for pertussis during the first six months of life.

PERTUSSIS IN AFRICA

Epidemiology

Prior to large-scale vaccination in the 1970s, whooping cough may have been among the top 10 causes of death among infants and children in sub-Saharan Africa. However, because of the difficulty in diagnosing pertussis by using verbal autopsies, we cannot be sure of its true importance. Even in the United States, pertussis cases are widely unrecognized (Hinman et al., 1986). In Africa, as in other developing countries, pertussis mortality rates are highest in the first six months of life and decline rapidly with age. The age pattern of deaths differs from that of measles, from which death rarely occurs before 4 months of age.

Much of what is known about pertussis in Africa is based on two longitudinal studies conducted in rural areas—Machakos, Kenya, and Niakhar, Senegal. In Machakos, two epidemics of pertussis occurred between 1974 and 1981. The average annual incidence for the period 1974-1981 was estimated at 1.6 percent among children under age 15 and 2.7 percent among children under age 5. Vaccination coverage was relatively low during this period. The case-fatality rate was 10 per 1,000 for all ages combined and 26 per 1,000 under age 1 (Muller et al., 1984b). These case-fatality rates (like the rates for measles in Machakos) are much lower than those recorded elsewhere (World Health Organization, 1975).

The pertussis incidence rate in Niakhar between 1983 and 1986 was 107 per 1,000 among children under age 5. The median age of cases was

4.5 years, and vaccination coverage was very low during this period (4 percent). However, as vaccination coverage increased between 1987 and 1989, the incidence rate was reduced by 79 percent (M. Garenne, personal communication, 1992). The case-fatality rates between 1983 and 1986 were 23 per 1,000 for all ages combined and 59 per 1,000 for infants. During 1987-1989, when vaccination coverage was higher and children were treated whenever possible, the case-fatality rate among children under 5 dropped to 13 per 1,000, a reduction of 43 percent. There were no pertussis deaths in the study area between 1988 and 1990 (Garenne et al., 1991). Cases of malnutrition were observed twice as often among children under age 5 after pertussis as after measles (Garenne and Cantrelle, 1986).

Vaccine Efficacy

In Machakos, the incidence of pertussis among vaccinated children was 54 percent lower than among nonrandomized controls of the same birth cohorts (Muller et al., 1984a,b). This finding suggests a vaccine efficacy similar to that observed in developed countries. Similar values were also found in South Africa. Investigation of an epidemic in Cape Town, South Africa, in 1988-1989 (Strebel et al., 1991) estimated an incidence rate of 66.7 percent among pre-primary school children with less than two doses of the DPT vaccine and 32.1 percent among those with three or four doses of the vaccine. This incidence suggests an efficacy of the pertussis vaccine of 52 percent (95 percent C.I. 12-74 percent). Preliminary results of a study conducted in Senegal showed a similar efficacy of 65 percent (M. Garenne, personal communication, 1992). Much of the variation in the vaccine efficacy arises from a range of case definitions. If a case definition of three weeks of cough is used, then the vaccine will have a high efficacy; but if a case definition of the presence of bacteria and one day of cough is used, the vaccine efficacy will be lower.

PROGRAM EFFORT

Figure 3-4 shows the proportion of children aged 12-23 months who had received three DPT injections as recorded in surveys taken around 1981 and 1991. In 1981, about 21-24 percent of African children had received three DPT injections (United Nations Children's Fund, 1991). By 1991 the proportion had increased to about 50 percent (International Science and Technology Institute, 1990; Expanded Programme on Immunization, 1992; Nigerian Federal Office of Statistics and Institute for Resource Development, 1992). This increase shows substantial progress, but leaves many children unprotected. The average for the continent is heavily influenced by low coverage rates in the three largest countries in the region. For 1991,

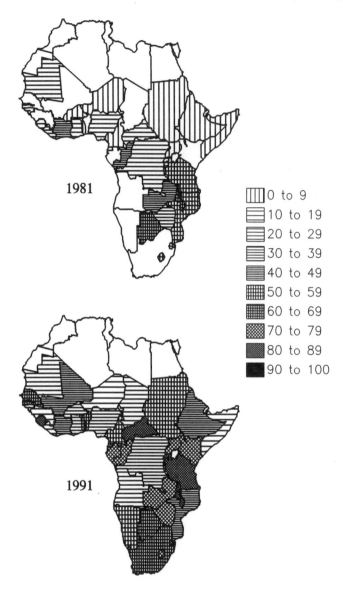

FIGURE 3-4 Proportions of children aged 12-23 months who have received three injections of DPT vaccine, countries of sub-Saharan Africa, 1981 and 1991. SOURCES: 1981 data from United Nations Children's Fund (1991); 1991 data from International Science and Technology Institute (1990) and Expanded Programme on Immunization (1992).

Nigeria had a rate of 33 percent, Ethiopia 44 percent, and Zaire 32 percent. In the rest of the region, coverage averaged 60 percent. However, the coverage rates in any one country can change drastically from year to year in response to major vaccination campaigns and political disturbances.

Unlike measles, there are very few studies of trends in the incidence of reported cases of pertussis. Data on outpatient cases of pertussis and coverage with three injections of DPT are available for Malawi between 1976 and 1987, as shown in Figure 3-5 (Expanded Programme on Immunization, 1989). During most of the period, vaccination coverage was increasing and the number of cases tended to decline. However, there were relatively large numbers of cases reported in the last three years of the series, which may have been due to the number of unvaccinated older children. The correlation between coverage and incidence is only .28, not statistically significant. However, in Cape Town, South Africa, pertussis death rates among nonwhites declined dramatically after introduction of the DPT vaccine in January 1950 (Strebel et al., 1991).

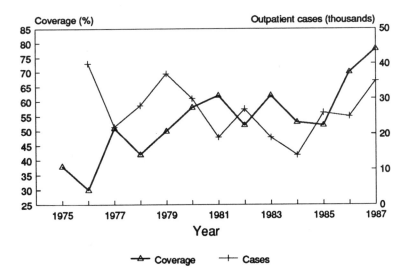

FIGURE 3-5 Trends in pertussis vaccination coverage and reported cases of pertussis in Malawi, 1976-1987. NOTE: Pertussis vaccination coverage is defined as children having three doses of vaccination against diphtheria, pertussis, and tetanus. SOURCE: Expanded Programme on Immunization (1989).

SUMMARY

Pertussis receives relatively little attention because it is less visible than other diseases and its symptoms are less distinguishable from those of other diseases. The pertussis vaccine, requiring at least three doses to be effective, is an essential component of child survival programs. The exact effect of the pertussis component of EPI vaccination on child mortality has not yet been determined, although studies suggest a wide range of efficacy. As with measles, a major benefit of the pertussis vaccine is that it lowers the severity of infection. As a consequence, it is also likely to lower the incidence of malnutrition, which is often caused by severe whooping cough. Immunization coverage has improved in recent years and is currently estimated at approximately 50 percent.

Case management currently includes treatment with antibiotics, although the disease is seldom detected when therapy can be most effective. Strategies for the most appropriate case management of whooping cough in the population require further research.

TUBERCULOSIS AND LEPROSY

Tuberculosis may be responsible for more deaths worldwide than any other disease caused by a single pathogen (Sudre et al., 1992). Approximately 171 million Africans are infected with tuberculosis; the prevalence rate is about 34 percent (Sudre et al., 1992). The annual incidence rate of 2.65 per 1,000 population is the highest of all regions. About one-sixth of these new cases are in individuals who are infected with the human immunodeficiency virus, which causes AIDS. The annual mortality rate due to tuberculosis is about 0.9 to 1.0 per 1,000 population—also higher than in any other region of the world. Only about 15 percent of tuberculosis cases occur in the population under age 15. The largest proportion of cases is found among adults aged 25 to 44 years (Murray, 1991).

Because the vaccination for tuberculosis also prevents leprosy, we consider that disease here as well. Its incidence and epidemiology are discussed later.

EPIDEMIOLOGY OF TUBERCULOSIS

In children, infection with the *Mycobacterium tuberculosis* is usually relatively benign and self-limiting. However, serious complications (particularly miliary disease—the presence of small nodules in the affected organ or body part—and tuberculous meningitis) are often fatal if left undiagnosed and untreated. Most diagnosed cases are in adults (Rodrigues,

1991), although many of these are the result of resurgence of infections acquired at earlier ages.

Data on causes of death among children rarely include tuberculosis, probably because of the difficulty of diagnosis. Verbal autopsies rarely provide a definitive diagnosis of tuberculosis, although cough lasting more than three months and weight loss are usually good indicators of respiratory tuberculosis. It is difficult to diagnosis pediatric tuberculosis even in clinics because of the difficulty in obtaining sputum samples from children and the unavailability of x-ray facilities. Moreover, the clinical symptoms of pediatric tuberculosis are often atypical, and tuberculin tests are difficult to interpret (Migliori et al., 1992). In addition, the mortality rate due to tuberculosis probably understates the likely effect of tuberculosis on child mortality because cases of tuberculosis may lead to severe weight loss and indirectly increase child mortality in other ways.

The tuberculosis situation in Africa is likely to worsen significantly during the next decade because of the link between AIDS and tuberculosis. The decline of an HIV patient's immunity often leads to the development of an overt infectious case of tuberculosis. Thus, the number of tuberculosis cases is increased through resurgence of old cases among HIV-positive individuals and through their spread of the disease to HIV-negative individuals. The incidence of tuberculosis among children will therefore increase in areas where HIV prevalence is high because even HIV-negative children will be subjected to an additional risk of infection. Schulzer et al. (1992) have projected that the annual risk of tuberculosis infection in HIV-negative individuals could increase by 13 to 141 percent in African countries, depending on the prevalence of tuberculosis and AIDS. In southern Uganda, the annual risk of smear-positive tuberculosis (i.e., infective cases capable of being transmitted) among HIV-negative adults could reach 0.4 percent by the year 2000. For the total population, Schulzer et al. estimate that the annual risk of infection could approach 2 percent per year. An increase in tuberculosis is already apparent in Tanzania, where the reported number of smear-positive cases increased from 8,000 in 1984 to 10,000 in 1989. In Uganda the annual number of confirmed cases doubled between 1984 and 1987 (Schulzer et al., 1992).

PREVENTION AND TREATMENT OF TUBERCULOSIS

There are two basic public health approaches to tuberculosis. The first is vaccination with bacille Calmette-Guérin. BCG was derived from a strain of *Mycobacterium bovis* and has been used as a vaccine against *M. tuberculosis* since the 1920s. In Africa, tuberculosis is also caused by *M. africanum*. BCG also provides some protection against *M. leprae*, which causes leprosy. It is now a central part of the Expanded Programme on Immunization.

In Africa, most pediatric tuberculosis cases result from transmission from an infectious case in an adult. Most active cases among adults result from reactivation of infections that may have been dormant for many years. Thus, the BCG immunization is not an effective means of reducing the incidence of tuberculosis because it does not protect against primary infection. The immunization merely reduces the risk of progression from latent infection to clinically active disease (Rieder, 1992). Therefore, the best approach to reducing incidence is treatment of cases to reduce the period of transmission. Drug therapy can cure tuberculosis and thereby prevent death from tuberculosis as well as reduce the spread of the disease. About 75 percent of cases requiring treatment are among those aged 15-59 (Murray et al., 1991), and these are the source of infection for most new cases.

The main problem in treatment programs is compliance because treatment lasts between 6 and 18 months. Patients often feel well long before they are cured, which leads to a high default rate. For example, in a program in northern Ghana, 52 percent of male and 40 percent of female patients did not complete their treatment (van der Werf et al., 1990). The default rates for the standard therapy were 24 percent and 16 percent, respectively, for programs in Mozambique and Tanzania (Murray et al., 1991). Default rates are lower in programs that utilize the more expensive "short-course" treatments. In Mozambique, Tanzania, and Malawi, default rates for short-course regimens were 11, 10, and 2 percent, respectively (Murray et al., 1991). When patients discontinue treatment before they are cured, they are at risk of a resurgence of the infection and are infectious for a longer period.

Murray et al. (1991) estimate the effective cure rates[5] of standard therapy in the national programs of Mozambique and Tanzania to be 66 and 60 percent, respectively. They estimate that the effectiveness of short-course therapy is about 90 percent in Malawi and Mozambique, and 86 percent in Tanzania.

High default rates encourage the development of drug-resistant strains. A study in northern Ghana (van der Werf et al., 1989) found that initial resistance (i.e., resistance among patients who reported that they had not received previous treatment) was 27 percent to the drug isoniazid, 23 percent to streptomycin, and 29 percent to thiacetazone. Only 45 percent of samples were sensitive to all three drugs. A study of trends in initial drug resistance in black adult patients in South Africa (Weyer and Kleeberg, 1992) showed that resistance to isoniazid declined from 29 percent in 1965-1970 to 14 percent in 1980-1988. Similarly, resistance to streptomycin dropped from 34 to 12 percent. These declines are probably a result of

---

[5]This rate includes an estimate of the proportion of defaulters that are cured.

improved treatment practices. However, drug resistance is still a problem in South Africa among some ethnic groups. For example, among the Xhosa, 23 percent of infections were resistant to isoniazid.

The studies of tuberculosis treatment programs have focused on the effectiveness of treatment among identified cases. Because there are probably large differences in the success of programs in identifying cases, it is difficult to estimate the effect of treatment programs on populations. In addition, most of the patients in treatment programs are adults. For these reasons, we limit our review to studies of the effectiveness of vaccination programs that provide BCG.

EFFICACY OF BACILLE CALMETTE-GUÉRIN (BCG) VACCINATION

Estimates of the efficacy of BCG in preventing tuberculosis vary from zero to 80 percent in numerous studies (Fine, 1988). During the past 30 years there has been extensive debate over the reasons for this variation. However, there is still no consensus on what factors lead to high efficacy. As a result, there is a need for studies to determine whether BCG is effective in numerous different populations. Although the efficacy of BCG in preventing tuberculosis is variable, the consensus is that it is efficacious—as high as 95 percent—in reducing the incidence of serious forms of tuberculosis, including miliary tuberculosis and tuberculous meningitis (Tuberculosis Control Programme and Expanded Programme on Immunization, 1986; Schwoebel et al., 1993). These complications, which are frequent in children, are usually fatal if left untreated. Uncomplicated cases among children are relatively benign but may be important underlying causes of mortality, working particularly through malnutrition.

BCG Efficacy Against Tuberculosis in Africa

There are three studies of the efficacy of BCG in preventing tuberculosis in Africa. All three are case-control studies that compare the vaccination history of tuberculosis cases with the history of nontubercular controls. There are numerous problems that can bias case-control studies (e.g., ascertainment of vaccination status and diagnosis of tuberculosis in children). However, the costs of randomized control trials are so high that it is not possible to carry out such studies in all regions (Smith, 1988).

Blin et al. (1986) carried out a case-control study of the efficacy of BCG in preventing tuberculosis. The cases were adults aged 17-26 who were newly diagnosed with sputum-positive pulmonary tuberculosis in 1983-1984 in the only tuberculosis dispensary in Yaoundé, Cameroon. Many of these cases were probably infected as children. The controls were from an antivenereal dispensary in Yaoundé and general dispensaries in two towns in the region. Vaccination status was determined by the presence or absence of a BCG residual scar. The subjects were between 0 and 18 years of age during the BCG mass vaccination campaign.[6] The estimated protective effect of BCG against pulmonary tuberculosis in young adults was 66 percent (95 percent C.I. 53-75 percent). This estimate controls for potential confounding by sex, age, socioeconomic group, and geographic region of origin. However, none of these variables was significantly related to differences in efficacy.

Tidjani et al. (1986) reported on a trial conducted in Togo of BCG among children age 6 years or less who were in contact with newly diagnosed cases of tuberculosis. These children were at increased risk of infection and therefore provided an efficient sample for measuring vaccine efficacy. The estimate of efficacy of BCG from this study is 66 percent (95 percent C.I. 54-74 percent). The data suggest that the efficacy is higher for more severe forms of the disease. Statistical controls for the closeness of contact with a case of tuberculosis (parents or others) and for age and sex reduce the estimated efficacy to close to 60 percent. However, the efficacy of BCG might be lower in this sample than in the general population because the subjects were exposed to higher doses of the bacteria, which could overwhelm the resistance they acquired from BCG.

The population of a case-control study initially conducted in Malawi between 1980 and 1984 by Fine et al. (1986) remained under observation through 1989 (Pönnighaus et al., 1992). (The original study is discussed in the following section with other studies of the efficacy of BCG vaccine against leprosy.) By the end of the 1989 follow-up, 180 new incident cases of tuberculosis had been diagnosed in the population of 83,445. Confirmation of tuberculosis was based on sputum specimens of self-reported cases collected at health centers and the district hospital. The infection rates among BCG scar-positive and BCG scar-negative individuals were very similar. The differences between the age-corrected estimates, based on a number of age groups, case definitions, and estimation techniques, were not significant. This finding suggests that BCG vaccination is not protective against tuberculosis in the population.

EPIDEMIOLOGY OF LEPROSY

Leprosy is an infectious disease caused by *Mycobacterium leprae*; it is rarely fatal. The individual's response to the infection depends on the

---

[6]From 1968 to 1976 the campaigns applied to the population up to age 20. After 1976, only newborn infants were vaccinated.

cellular immune mechanism. A person with a good cellular immune response is more likely to have a milder tuberculoid type, and a person with weak or no cellular immunity is likely to develop the lepromatous type (Bloom and Godol, 1983). The clinical symptoms vary from a single hypopigmented skin patch that heals spontaneously to damage to the nervous system, bones, eyes, muscles, and extremities. The average incubation period is estimated to be 2 to 4 years, though it may vary from 9 months to 12 years (World Health Organization, 1985). The World Health Organization (1982) recommends that treatment last between six months and two years, depending on the type of case. It is estimated that approximately 11.5 million cases of leprosy exist worldwide—5.3 million of which are registered for treatment (Irgens and Skjaerven, 1985). In Africa, it is thought that 3.5 million cases of leprosy exist. Only about 1 percent of the cases are estimated to be among children under age 5 (World Health Organization, 1982).

BCG also provides protection against leprosy, and this protection is an important element in the evaluation of its effect in Africa (Rieder, 1992). BCG provides some protection against leprosy through cross protection between *Mycobacterium bovis* and *M. leprae*. Studies of the efficacy of BCG against leprosy in Asia show it to be 20 percent efficacious in Myanmar, 30 percent in South India, and 44 percent in New Guinea (Fine and Pönnighaus, 1988).

There have been two studies of the efficacy of BCG in preventing leprosy in Africa. The first, conducted by Stanley et al. (1981), was a cohort study of children who were contacts or relatives of known leprosy patients in Uganda. In the first stage of the study in 1960-1962, 16,150 tuberculin-negative or weakly tuberculin-positive children were allocated at random to BCG-vaccinated and unvaccinated groups. The researchers examined these children at intervals of approximately two years for the next eight years. Eighty percent of these children were under age 10 at the start of the study. At the first follow-up visit in 1963, 1,976 children born into the trial families were added to the cohort to increase the number of young children in the study. Between 1970 and 1975, new cases at leprosy clinics were checked to see if they were included in the cohort study.

Stanley et al. estimated that the efficacy of BCG against leprosy was 80 percent (95 percent C.I. 72-86 percent) based on the experience of the original cohort recruited in 1960-1962 through 1970. The data from 1970 to 1975 suggest that the vaccine continued to be effective 12 to 13 years after vaccination. Data on the children who had lesions of doubtful etiology at intake suggested that BCG may not have had a large effect on preexisting leprosy lesions. However, the numbers of such cases were too small to produce reliable estimates of efficacy in slowing progression of the disease. Similarly, there was no evidence that BCG slowed the progression or severity of the disease in children who had no sign of lesions at intake (i.e., among apparent cases of vaccine failures).

Fine et al. (1986) ran a study of BCG efficacy against leprosy in northern Malawi. This study began with a survey of 112,000 households between 1980 and 1984. Each case of leprosy was matched with all individuals living in the same square kilometer who were of the same sex, five-year age group, and schooling status. The study was limited to those under age 35 because BCG coverage beyond that age was very low. Persons whose BCG scar status was doubtful or unknown (10.3 percent) were excluded from the analysis. Analysis of the matched case-control data led to an estimate of BCG efficacy against leprosy of 41 percent (95 percent C.I. 11-61 percent), showing very little difference across age groups. Data on cases of leprosy identified after the initial survey (i.e., through prospective data collection) led to an estimate of efficacy of 57 percent (95 percent C.I. 24-75 percent). The estimate of efficacy based on the case-control design (41 percent) was probably biased downward because it included some cases in which infection occurred before vaccination. Because of this bias and because errors in BCG scar ascertainment and in diagnosis of leprosy might reduce the efficacy estimate, the authors concluded that the efficacy was at least 50 percent. In a follow-up study between 1985 and 1989 among the same population, an efficacy of 50 percent or greater was observed (Pönnighaus et al., 1992).

These studies suggest that BCG is more effective against leprosy in Africa than in South India and Myanmar (Fine, 1988; Fine and Pönnighaus, 1988). There is no generally accepted explanation for this difference. However, it does appear that BCG is effective against leprosy in eastern and southern Africa. Because there are a large number of cases of leprosy in Nigeria, it would be useful to estimate the efficacy of the vaccine in that country.

PROGRAM COVERAGE

Figure 3-6 presents the estimates of coverage of BCG by country in 1981 and 1991 (Boerma et al., 1990; International Science and Technology Institute, 1990; United Nations Children's Fund, 1991; Expanded Programme on Immunization, 1992; Nigerian Federal Office of Statistics and Institute for Resource Development, 1992). For all of sub-Saharan Africa, BCG coverage increased from about 31-34 percent in 1981 to 72 percent in 1991. These estimates are very rough. Many of the estimates come from administrative records rather than population surveys. Even the data based on surveys usually have a 95 percent confidence interval of about ±10 percentage points. However, it is clear that BCG coverage has increased drastically during the past decade.

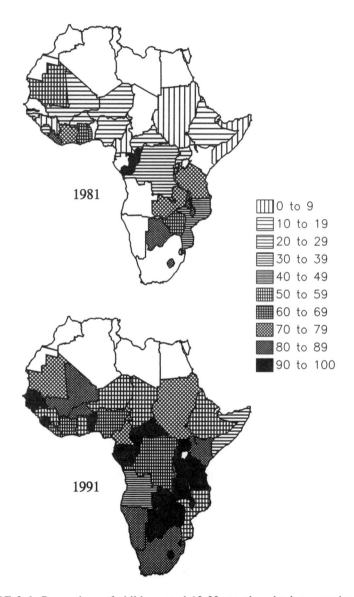

1981

1991

```
0 to 9
10 to 19
20 to 29
30 to 39
40 to 49
50 to 59
60 to 69
70 to 79
80 to 89
90 to 100
```

FIGURE 3-6 Proportions of children aged 12-23 months who have received BCG vaccination, countries of sub-Saharan Africa, 1981 and 1991. SOURCES: 1981 data from United Nations Children's Fund (1991); 1991 data from International Science and Technology Institute (1990) and Expanded Programme on Immunization (1992).

SUMMARY

The prevalence of tuberculosis in Africa is estimated to be 34 percent. Given the link between AIDS and tuberculosis, it is likely that the prevalence of tuberculosis will continue to increase. The BCG vaccination, although of varying and questionable efficacy, has been shown to be effective against both tuberculosis and leprosy in Africa. However, given the great variation in efficacy across continents, it would be useful to have more studies in different African settings.

Programs that provide BCG have probably saved many lives and reduced morbidity. However, no precise estimates of the effect of BCG on mortality exist. Childhood deaths that have tuberculosis as an underlying cause may actually outnumber the deaths directly attributed to the disease. Therefore, it is not possible to produce an accurate estimate of the likely effect of the increase in BCG coverage on child mortality in Africa.

TETANUS

Tetanus is a major cause of neonatal death in much of Africa, as well as among other age groups. Because of the small proportion of the population protected by immunization at all but childhood ages, and the large proportion of births that occur under poor hygienic conditions related especially to home deliveries, tetanus mortality rates in Africa are probably among the highest in the world. The tetanus mortality rate is best documented for neonates—the population in which the problem predominates. Tetanus of the umbilicus is responsible for a substantial proportion of neonatal and infant mortality in many regions where most deliveries are performed by untrained traditional birth attendants or relatives.

EPIDEMIOLOGY

The few available studies suggest that rates of 10 to 20 neonatal tetanus deaths per 1,000 live births are not unusual. Studies in rural parts of Sierra Leone have led to estimates as high as 70 per 1,000 (Kandeh, 1986). Tetanus may be less of a problem in southern and eastern Africa than in western Africa. The Machakos project in Kenya recorded a rate of only 1.2 per 1,000 (van Ginneken and Muller, 1984).

Some studies of tetanus are apparently biased by underreporting of neonatal deaths. This bias is particularly important for estimates based on retrospective reporting of deaths. In several studies, underreporting is apparent in the trends of tetanus mortality rates. In particular, several surveys show higher rates for the months closer to the survey date (e.g., Stanfield and Galazka (1984) and Sokal et al. (1988) in Côte d'Ivoire; Expanded Programme on Immunization (1983) in Malawi; however, Melgaard et al. (1988) report no trend in Kenya). On the other hand, estimates of tetanus mortality may be biased upward by errors in diagnosis. For example, Snow et al. (1992) compared verbal autopsies with records of hospital deaths. They found that verbal autopsies performed rather well for neonatal tetanus deaths (sensitivity of 90 percent and specificity of 79 percent). These led to an exaggeration of the neonatal tetanus mortality rate of about 30 percent.

More sophisticated treatment of tetanus cases is not currently a viable policy option because such treatment is expensive and difficult. The case-fatality rate of hospitalized cases of neonatal tetanus is usually 60-80 percent (Bwibo, 1971; Kenya Ministry of Health, 1978; Merhai and Kumar, 1986; Maru et al., 1988; Babaniyi and Parakoyi, 1989; Einterz and Bates, 1991). There are fewer data on tetanus after the first month of life. In Kenya in 1978, the case-fatality rate among inpatient cases was 33 percent for children 1-14 and 47 percent for adults over age 15 (Kenya Ministry of Health, 1978).

A study in Tanzania reported a lower case-fatality rate among neonates treated with antitetanus equine serum (Mongi et al., 1987). However, a recent meta-analysis (which included the study by Mongi et al.) did not find convincing evidence that this approach improved survival among neonates with tetanus (Abrutyn and Berlin, 1991). Yet, the effect of serum depends on when it is given. During the first two days of life, it has a beneficial effect; thereafter, it does not (M. Garenne, personal communication, 1992).

Although improvements in case fatality are possible, only a small proportion of neonatal cases ever receive hospital treatment (Expanded Programme on Immunization, 1983; Babaniyi and Parakoyi, 1989). For example, in a rural area of Côte d'Ivoire, only 2 percent of neonatal tetanus cases came to the attention of medical authorities (Sokal et al., 1988). During 1979 in Kenya, there were 2,258 outpatient cases and 767 inpatient cases of tetanus at all ages in the 33 districts for which data were available (Kenya Ministry of Health, 1978). Extrapolating to the whole population, the Ministry of Health estimated that there were about 3,300 cases at all ages nationally. In comparison, Melgaard et al. (1988) used data on three districts to estimate that there were about 8,000 to 12,000 neonatal deaths due to tetanus annually in the mid-1980s. It is likely therefore that only a fraction of cases of tetanus ever receive even minimal care.

PROGRAMS TO REDUCE THE INCIDENCE OF NEONATAL TETANUS

In 1989 the World Health Assembly called for the worldwide elimination of neonatal tetanus by 1995 (World Health Organization, 1990). The two policy options are improving delivery practices and providing immunizations. One way to improve deliveries is to increase the proportion of deliveries that occur in hospitals or dispensaries where it is easier to maintain appropriate antiseptic practices. In hospitals and dispensaries, it is also possible to administer tetanus antitoxin to newborns shortly after delivery—a practice common in francophone areas (Sokal et al., 1988). Alihonou (1970) attributes the rapid decline or reported deaths from neonatal tetanus in Dakar to this practice. An alternative approach is to train traditional birth attendants or midwives to improve home deliveries by using sterile instruments for cutting the umbilicus and to treat the stump appropriately.

The other option is immunization of pregnant women, which provides temporary immunity to the fetus and protects the newborn for several months. The World Health Organization recommendation is that women receive two injections of tetanus toxoid at least one month apart as early as possible during pregnancy. One study (Owa and Makinde, 1990) suggests that children who do contract neonatal tetanus have a greater chance of survival if their mother has had a single prenatal tetanus injection. A single booster injection is recommended for subsequent pregnancies. Four or five tetanus toxoid vaccinations are likely to provide lifetime protection for the mother and for each of her children during the neonatal period (Wassilak and Berlin, 1986). In areas where neonatal tetanus is a serious problem, vaccination programs should target all women of childbearing age.

In practice, most programs include efforts both to improve deliveries and to provide tetanus immunization to women. Although the combination is probably more efficacious than either approach alone, it is difficult to evaluate the independent efficacy of each approach. Only one study has attempted to compare these strategies. Orenstein et al. (1985, quoted in Babaniyi and Parakoyi, 1989), estimated that in Nigeria the efficacy of two doses of tetanus toxoid was higher than that of either hospital delivery or home delivery by a trained midwife.

Incidence of Neonatal Tetanus Among Hospital Deliveries

Several studies have shown that the incidence of neonatal tetanus is much lower among hospital deliveries than among other births (Dan et al., 1971; Stanfield and Galazka, 1984; Kofoed and Simonsen, 1988; Sokal et al., 1988). Melgaard et al. (1987) reported that in three districts of Kenya the neonatal tetanus mortality rates were 14.1 for home deliveries and 4.3 for deliveries in health institutions. These estimates yield a relative risk of 3.3 associated with home deliveries compared to hospital deliveries. Other studies have found that all recorded cases of neonatal tetanus were among children born at home (e.g., Sokal et al., 1988).

Women who deliver in hospitals may be different from other women in many ways (e.g., they are more likely to live in urban areas and may be better educated). However, the lower incidence of neonatal tetanus among hospital births also probably reflects better care of the umbilical stump. Even so, hospital delivery is not a guarantee of protection. Even the most careful delivery will not protect the child against treatment of the stump or circumcision practices after the child leaves the hospital.

Evidence of the Effect of Training of Traditional Birth Attendants

Because of the high cost and unavailability of hospital deliveries for most African women in rural areas, many authorities have recommended training traditional birth attendants (TBAs) in aseptic procedures for cutting the umbilical cord and caring for the umbilical stump. A study by Leroy and Garenne (1991) in rural Senegal suggests that the most important risk factor for neonatal tetanus is whether or not the person who delivered the baby washed her hands with soap prior to cutting the cord. However, most training programs have concentrated on improving the instrument used for cutting the cord.

There are very few studies anywhere in the world that provide evidence of the effect of training TBAs on tetanus mortality in populations in which tetanus toxoid coverage did not also increase (Ross, 1986). Studies in the Philippines and Bangladesh have shown that midwife training reduces overall neonatal mortality more than maternal immunization, but maternal immunization alone causes a larger reduction in the incidence of neonatal tetanus than midwife training (Stanfield and Galazka, 1984).

There has been one such study in Africa in the Thies region of Senegal. In the first part of the study, birth attendants in six villages learned to care for the cord properly. After this training, the neonatal mortality rate in the program villages was 38 per 1,000 live births, compared to 101 in the control villages (Dan et al., 1971). The recorded postneonatal rates in the two areas were identical (147 and 146 per 1,000).

In the years following this study, the program reached an increasing number of villages. Sanokho and Senghor (1975, quoted by Ross, 1986) examined the place of residence of neonatal tetanus cases recorded at the Khombole hospital. The proportion of these cases that were from villages selected for the midwife training program dropped substantially after the start of the program. These studies suggest that the training of traditional birth attendants can reduce the incidence of neonatal tetanus, at least in populations with high rates.

Evidence of the Effect of Programs that Provide Tetanus Toxoid Immunization to Women

Studies of antenatal immunization against tetanus in other parts of the world have shown that two injections of tetanus toxoid early in pregnancy are 95 percent effective in preventing neonatal tetanus in the child born of that pregnancy. The effect of two injections declines over time. Some studies show that the injections are still 40 percent effective in reducing neonatal tetanus four to five years later, and Koenig (1992) reports that two doses of tetanus toxoid may provide protection against neonatal tetanus for 15 years or more. A single booster shot restores the full effectiveness. A single injection during pregnancy provides partial protection for that pregnancy (see summary in Stanfield and Galazka, 1984).

Susceptibility to tetanus and case-fatality rates are not affected by the presence of other common diseases (e.g., malaria, malnutrition). Therefore, there is no reason to expect that at a given level of neonatal tetanus mortality and a given level of program coverage, the effect of an immunization program would differ across populations. What is uncertain is the success rate of various types of programs in achieving high levels of effective coverage. In particular, there is little information on the proportion of women who deliver at home after receiving at least two injections of tetanus toxoid. We also do not have studies that suggest what proportion of births are partially protected by tetanus toxoid injections during a previous pregnancy.

A few studies in Africa have demonstrated the efficacy of immunization with or without midwife training programs. Ross (1986) reported the results of a program that formed village health teams in 11 villages near Serabu Hospital, Sierra Leone. The program trained TBAs in improved perinatal care and encouraged them to refer pregnant women for antenatal care, which included tetanus toxoid injections. Within a year of the start of the program, the neonatal tetanus mortality rate declined from 72 to 11 per 1,000 live births (this difference is significant at the 0.001 level). In the next few years, the mortality from neonatal tetanus continued to decline to "virtually zero" (Ross, 1986). The program near Serabu Hospital must be considered a field trial because it is not clear whether that program could be successfully replicated in larger populations.

Two studies of large-scale programs that participated in the Combatting Childhood Communicable Diseases (CCCD) project, funded by the U.S. Agency for International Development and carried out by the Centers for Disease Control of the U.S. Department of Health and Human Services, provide some evidence of the efficacy of tetanus immunization on neonatal mortality. In one area of Zaire and two counties in Liberia, the CCCD programs were evaluated by using retrospective maternity histories before and after the start of the program. In Liberia, data on cause of death based on verbal autopsies suggested that there was a reduction of approximately 50 percent in neonatal tetanus mortality (probability less than .05; Becker et al., 1993). This decrease was probably the result of an increase in the proportion of mothers who had received two tetanus toxoid injections from very low levels to more than 30 percent (Vernon et al., 1993). The CCCD surveys in Zaire did not include verbal autopsies. However, there was no evidence of a decline in infant mortality. This apparent lack of effect is consistent with the absence of neonatal tetanus cases reported by the local hospital and health centers before the program (Vernon et al., 1993).

Because case-fatality rates are so high and few cases receive modern medical care, we can safely use data on disease incidence to monitor programs. A study of neonatal tetanus in Maputo, Mozambique, suggests that a vaccination program alone can have a significant effect in urban areas. Cutts et al. (1990b) reported that from 1976 to 1978, there were between 173 and 254 cases of neonatal tetanus reported annually in Maputo. After the start of the vaccination campaign, the proportion of mothers reporting at least two injections of tetanus toxoid increased to 42 percent in 1982, 91 percent in 1983, and 87 percent in 1986. This increase in vaccination coverage coincided with a rapid decline in the number of reported cases to a range of only 3 to 13 cases per year between 1982 and 1987. Although it is not possible to calculate the mortality effect of this program based on these surveillance data, the program must have been associated with a dramatic drop in neonatal tetanus mortality.

In Malawi, immunization of pregnant women with tetanus toxoid began in 1984. Coverage increased from about 27 percent in 1985 to more than 60 percent in 1988[7] (Expanded Programme on Immunization, 1989). Although the number of neonatal tetanus cases reported in hospitals dropped in 1986 and 1987, the change was not significant.

Finally, Sokal et al. (1988) quoted a study by Yada et al. (1981) from Burkina Faso. In one area of the country, coverage with two injections of tetanus toxoid reached 50 percent and hospital admissions for tetanus decreased by two-thirds.

PROGRAM COVERAGE

Figure 3-7 presents national estimates for 1981 and 1991 of the proportion of recent deliveries in which the woman had at least two injections of tetanus toxoid during pregnancy (International Science and Technology Institute, 1990; United Nations Children's Fund, 1991; Expanded Programme on Immunization, 1992; Nigerian Federal Office of Statistics and Institute for Resource Development, 1992). In 1991, about 41 percent of deliveries were protected by recent tetanus toxoid injections. This coverage is much larger than the value for 1981, which was less than 15 percent. Estimates for West Africa, where neonatal tetanus may be more common, indicate that

---

[7]These figures were read from the graph in the article.

coverage increased from about 12 to 44 percent. These estimates are subject to numerous types of sampling and reporting error because they are often based on women's retrospective reporting and on sample surveys. In addition, children born to women who received several tetanus toxoid injections during previous pregnancies are partially protected against tetanus. Despite these weaknesses, the data suggest substantial improvements in coverage, although most pregnancies are still not protected.

PROGRAMS TO REDUCE
NONNEONATAL TETANUS MORTALITY

The standard EPI program in most African countries includes tetanus immunization of young children as part of the DPT series. With the high coverage rates achieved in many areas, there have likely been reductions in nonneonatal and pediatric tetanus. However, to our knowledge there have not been any studies of the effect of this aspect of EPI programs. Similarly, antenatal immunization may have reduced tetanus mortality among adult women, but we are not aware of any studies of the effect of these programs on adult mortality.

SUMMARY

Tetanus is a leading cause of neonatal death in sub-Saharan Africa, with a range of 10 to 20 deaths per 1,000 live births in much of the region prior to control efforts. Lower rates in southern and eastern Africa suggest that regional differentials exist in neonatal mortality, but this result could be due to biases arising from underreporting of neonatal deaths. Programs designed to reduce mortality from neonatal tetanus generally focus on improving delivery conditions (such as training TBAs to incorporate sanitary practices) and immunizations of pregnant women or women of reproductive age.

A number of studies conducted in Liberia, Mozambique, and Burkina Faso indicate that as the proportion of pregnant women who are immunized increases, mortality from neonatal tetanus decreases. For a woman to be covered adequately against tetanus, she needs to have received at least two injections of tetanus toxoid at least one month apart as early as possible during the pregnancy (the first time she receives the immunization), with a single booster injection (up to three) given during subsequent pregnancies for the mother and for the child during the neonatal period. Results from the Demographic and Health Survey indicate that a relatively large proportion of mothers of children born during the five years prior to the survey in most countries were adequately immunized against tetanus. Similarly, an association is observed between women being immunized against tetanus

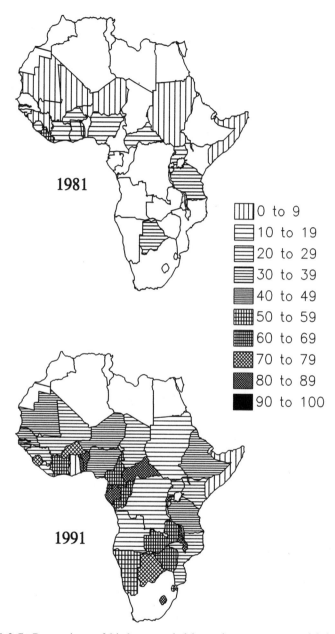

FIGURE 3-7 Proportions of births preceded by at least two prenatal injections of tetanus toxoid, countries of sub-Saharan Africa, 1981 and 1991. SOURCES: 1981 data from United Nations Children's Fund (1991); 1991 data from International Science and Technology Institute (1990) and Expanded Programme on Immunization (1992).

and those having hospital-based deliveries. Thus, the women with the greatest likelihood of having unsanitary conditions at delivery are also those who have not received adequate immunization against neonatal tetanus.

CONCLUSION

The Expanded Programme on Immunization has had a large impact on increasing vaccination coverage. As noted earlier, vaccination coverage for the preventable diseases included in the EPI increased substantially between the 1980s and 1990s, as illustrated by the increase in BCG coverage from 28 to 79 percent and measles vaccination coverage from 18 to 54 percent. Despite the increase in coverage, the quantity and quality of research on the effects of various components of standard EPI immunization programs on child mortality are uneven.

Measles has been studied widely in Africa from epidemiological and programmatic perspectives. Programs using the standard age schedule for vaccination with the standard vaccine can be effective in preventing measles and reducing child mortality in Africa by large proportions. Although the vaccine is highly efficacious, studies indicate that in some large-scale programs, cold chain failures have greatly reduced program effectiveness. In some study areas, program effectiveness has varied substantially over time. Although vaccination coverage is increasing, measles is not likely to be eliminated from Africa in the near future. Thus, in addition to the need for continued research on the disease's epidemiology, we need to know more about treatment strategies for children who contract the disease.

The vaccination coverage for pertussis has not achieved the EPI program goal of 75 percent; currently, it is estimated to be about 57 percent. Pertussis is difficult to diagnose because it has no uniquely distinguishing symptoms in its early stages. A wide range of estimates of the efficacy of the pertussis component of the DPT series has been reported. The vaccine, however, has reduced the incidence of the disease and may lower the severity of infection among those who are vaccinated and become ill. We do not have any estimates of the effect of DPT on mortality.

Tuberculosis is an important cause of mortality and morbidity among both children and adults in Africa, with an estimated prevalence of 34 percent. Its effect among children may be underestimated because it is often a contributing cause, rather than the primary cause of death. The BCG vaccination is of questionable efficacy in preventing cases of tuberculosis—estimates range from 0 to 80 percent—but may be more effective in preventing the more serious forms of the disease. It has also been shown to be effective in preventing leprosy.

Tetanus is a leading cause of neonatal mortality in some areas of sub-

Saharan Africa. It is preventable if the mother has been adequately vaccinated. Other options for reducing the disease are the training of traditional birth attendants in hygienic delivery practices and the administration of tetanus antitoxin to the child shortly after delivery.

Before the initiation of the Expanded Programme on Immunization, as recently as the early 1980s, vaccination coverage in Africa was the lowest in the world (Rodrigues, 1991). To augment national programs, acceleration strategies based on outreach components such as mobile units and improved cold chains were implemented in the mid-1980s. Greater attention to these preventable diseases through increased immunization has probably had a large effect on reducing mortality, but the full potential of these programs has not been achieved. Increased coverage with the standard EPI immunizations and maintenance of high coverage should continue to be top priorities for reducing child mortality.

4

Other Interventions Targeted
at Single Diseases

In addition to the diseases that can be prevented through immunization, there are other diseases that are responsible for large proportions of mortality in Africa. In this chapter, we examine diarrheal diseases, malaria, and acute respiratory infections.

Currently, programs aimed at controlling diarrheal diseases focus on a case-management strategy that promotes the use of oral rehydration therapy, which includes oral rehydration solutions, recommended home fluids such as rice water or gruels, and feeding with extra fluid. In addition, diarrheal disease control programs promote breastfeeding and safe weaning practices, use of potable water, and personal and domestic hygiene. Programs that combine these different strategies are in operation in almost all sub-Saharan African countries.

Malaria is a major cause of morbidity among children and adults, but is particularly serious among infants and children. Strategies for controlling malaria include eliminating breeding places for mosquitoes that transmit the disease, direct killing of mosquitoes with insecticide, preventing mosquito bites by means of barriers such as bed nets, drug prevention, and treating fevers that may be due to malaria.

Acute respiratory infections (ARIs) are also discussed in this chapter. Pneumonia is the principal cause of death among these diseases, although bronchitis, asthma, and influenza are also responsible for some infant and child deaths. The strategy promoted by the World Health Organization emphasizes early detection of these infections and appropriate antibiotic treatment made available through primary health care programs. Although these diseases are a major cause of infant and child deaths in the region, relatively few sub-Saharan African countries yet have national ARI control programs.

DIARRHEAL DISEASE CONTROL PROGRAMS

The term diarrheal diseases refers to a heterogeneous group of illnesses characterized by frequent loose or liquid stools and caused by a wide variety of viral and bacterial pathogens, as well as a few parasites. These conditions can also be classified as acute watery, dysenteric, or persistent diarrhea, according to their clinical presentation. Acute watery diarrhea can be associated with substantial losses of water and electrolytes, resulting in life-threatening dehydration. Although not the most important cause of acute dehydrating diarrhea in African children, cholera can also lead to high mortality in some settings. Cholera epidemics in the 1970s and 1980s had high case-fatality rates in many countries in sub-Saharan Africa (Glass and Black, 1992). Dysentery (generally defined as loose or liquid stools with blood) does not commonly result in dehydration and therefore is less often life threatening. It may require specific antimicrobial therapy. Persistent diarrhea, usually defined as any diarrheal episode that continues for 14 days or more, is often found in children who have malnutrition and a high incidence of prior diarrhea. Therapy is focused predominantly on nutritional management during and after the illness.

There is limited information on the frequency of occurrence of the various clinical syndromes of diarrhea or the frequency of dehydration. In The Gambia, it was found that 17 percent of children had at least one episode of clinically dehydrating diarrhea in the first two years of life (Goh-Rowland et al., 1985).

EPIDEMIOLOGY

Diarrheal diseases are recognized as an important public health problem in the countries of sub-Saharan Africa. A recent review by Kirkwood (1991) of more than 100 surveys or longitudinal studies of diarrheal disease in 33 sub-Saharan African countries found that the overall median incidence of diarrhea was 4.9 episodes per year for a child less than 5 years old, and that the median prevalence was nearly 10 percent. Where information was available by age, the peak rates of incidence and prevalence appeared to occur in children 6-18 months old, as in other developing countries. In sub-Saharan Africa, diarrhea is generally the most common cause of death during the postneonatal period and the second most common among children aged 1-4 years.

Globally, diarrheal diseases are considered to be one of the two leading causes of death among children. Again, as summarized by Kirkwood (1991), a large number of studies using various methodologies to ascertain the causes of death indicated that a median of 38 percent of all deaths in children aged 0-4 years were associated with diarrhea, but within a wide range from 4 to 70 percent. Studies of the diarrheal mortality rate among children under age 5 are infrequent, and many of the studies that exist are of questionable validity. It is very difficult to obtain reliable estimates of incidence rates even with frequent surveillance. For example, reliability tests in Kenya suggest that mothers were overreporting diarrhea among children by 15 to 40 percent (Leeuwenburg et al., 1978). Among the studies using better methodologies, estimates ranging from 3.4 to 18.0 diarrheal deaths annually per 1,000 children under 5 years old were found for small areas of Kenya, Malawi, Senegal, and Tanzania.

It has generally been believed that many if not most of the childhood deaths associated with diarrhea in developing countries are the result of acute dehydration. Undoubtedly acute dehydrating diarrhea represents a substantial proportion of the diarrheal deaths, but it may be less a predominant cause than initially believed. Recent information from four countries (India, Bangladesh, Brazil, and Senegal) indicates that acute watery diarrhea accounted for about 35 percent (25-46 percent) of all diarrhea-associated deaths (Programme for Control of Diarrhoeal Diseases, 1991a). In Bangladesh, 40 percent of diarrhea-associated deaths in the age group 1-11 months and only 9 percent in the age group 1-4 years had acute watery diarrhea (Fauveau et al., 1991). The remainder of the diarrhea-associated deaths in these settings were associated with either acute or persistent dysentery or persistent nondysenteric diarrhea. In 30 villages in Senegal, 46 percent of the diarrhea-associated deaths in children under 5 years of age were with acute diarrhea, 47 percent with persistent diarrhea, and 8 percent with dysentery. In addition to the role of diarrhea as a primary cause of death, it may also contribute indirectly to high mortality through malnutrition and micronutrient deficiency, which are important underlying factors for a high proportion of child mortality in sub-Saharan Africa.

Information on the epidemiology of diarrhea in Africa indicates great similarity with other impoverished populations in developing countries that have crowded conditions, inadequate sanitation, limited quantity and quality of water, and poor personal and domestic hygiene (Kirkwood, 1991). One major source of infection is weaning foods, which are often stored and fed to the child throughout the day (Rowland et al., 1978; van Steenbergen et al., 1983). As in the other settings, malnutrition is common, and some infectious diseases such as measles and malaria may also increase the incidence or adverse consequences of diarrhea.

TREATMENT

Diarrheal disease control programs in developing countries, including those in sub-Saharan Africa, have focused primarily on the management of acute dehydrating diarrhea (Claeson and Merson, 1990). Studies begun in the 1970s demonstrated that diarrheal dehydration could be treated with oral as opposed to intravenous fluid and electrolyte replacement, potentially making this therapy much more widely accessible (Parker et al., 1985). Subsequent studies have borne out the applicability of oral rehydration therapy (ORT), along with continued feeding in the management of diarrhea. This approach, with the selective use of intravenous fluids for severely dehydrated cases, has formed the mainstay of diarrheal disease control programs. Unfortunately, not much attention has been paid to date to protocols for the correct use of antibiotics for the treatment of dysentery or to the dietary management of persistent diarrhea, and these two problems may account for a majority of the diarrhea-associated deaths.

The efficacy of ORT in comparison with intravenous therapy has been amply demonstrated in controlled research settings throughout the last two decades. Furthermore, the effectiveness of ORT in hospitals (based on inpatients) has also been proven. Studies of children under age 5 in hospitals in Angola, Malawi, and Nigeria have documented declines of 39 to 95 percent in case-fatality rates among all diarrheal patients (World Health Organization, 1988). Studies in Angola, Nigeria, and Zaire further documented reductions in under-5 inpatient diarrheal case-fatality rates ranging from 7 to 46 percent (World Health Organization, 1988). In only one study in Malawi did the inpatient case-fatality rate increase; this result was linked to an increase in the severity of cases that were admitted to the hospital, with more patients being managed as outpatients. In addition to reducing case-fatality rates, ORT programs in these major hospitals reduced inpatient admissions by 10-95 percent, and in several cases, the average number of days children were kept in the hospital declined by more than a day.

Although there has not been a population-based study that demonstrates a reduction in mortality from the introduction of ORT in hospitals in Africa, there has been one in a rural area of Bangladesh. This study indicated that in an area with high access to a diarrheal treatment center, facility-based care may have reduced infant mortality by 1-8 percent and 1- to 4-year-old mortality by 4-14 percent (Oberle et al., 1990). Another study in the same area of rural Bangladesh also suggested that the diarrheal treatment center resulted in an 8 percent reduction in infant mortality and a 12 percent reduction in 1- to 4-year-old mortality (Chen et al., 1983).

It has been hypothesized that the use of oral rehydration therapy begun early in an episode of diarrhea could prevent the development of dehydration and reduce related mortality. A number of community-based research studies were conducted to evaluate the effect of home management of diarrhea on total and diarrhea-associated mortality. These studies are reviewed here briefly because they provide the only available evidence of the efficacy or effectiveness of diarrheal disease control programs in relation to mortality at a population level.

A study conducted between 1977 and 1979 in a remote area of Bangladesh compared mortality in a village in which oral rehydration solution was provided for episodes of diarrhea, with mortality in another village where persons had no home provision of treatment but were closer to a diarrheal treatment center than the treatment group (Rahaman et al., 1979). The study reported that the village with home ORT (78 percent of diarrheal episodes being treated) had a diarrheal mortality rate among infants of 1.6 per 1,000 compared to 17.4 per 1,000 population in the comparison area. The diarrheal mortality rate in children 1-4 years was 1.9 per 1,000 in the intervention area and 5.7 per 1,000 in the comparison area. Rahaman et al. (1982) compared the comparison group and other nonintervention areas and reported that the attendance rate at the diarrheal treatment center for persons living further away was lower. Also children living more than 2 miles away from the treatment center had higher diarrhea-associated mortality than those living closer to the center.

A number of studies have been conducted in Egypt, first as large-scale community-based intervention trials and later as evaluations of an extensive National Control of Diarrheal Diseases Program. A study begun in 1980 in the Nile Delta (Dakahlaia governorate) to compare various delivery strategies for oral rehydration therapy (Kielmann et al., 1985) described a decrease of 40 percent in total childhood mortality after the introduction of ORT through home visiting. A different intervention, also in the Nile Delta (Menoufia governorate), in the same time period did not succeed in substantially altering the diarrheal treatment practices in "treatment villages" compared with "control villages," and reported no change in childhood mortality rates (Tekçe, 1982).

The National Control of Diarrheal Diseases Program (NCDDP) in Egypt later achieved wide use of ORT for diarrhea of 50 percent and higher. After the program had been in operation for four years, the intervention and control areas involved in the previous Dakahlaia governorate study were evaluated for trends in mortality (National Control of Diarrheal Diseases Project, 1988). In 1986 the use of ORT was equivalent in what had previously been intervention and control areas as a result of national program efforts. By this time, there was no longer a difference in mortality rates, which in both instances were about half of those at the onset of the intervention study in 1980. Most of the mortality reduction was reported to be related to a drop in diarrhea-associated mortality. Further evaluation of the NCDDP has indicated substantial declines in infant mortality of approximately 8 per 1,000 and diarrhea-associated infant mortality of approximately 7 per 1,000 on a national basis (Rashad, 1989, 1992; El-Rafie et al., 1990). The temporal concordance of the sharp drops in mortality with the increasing rates of treatment with ORT, along with the apparent decrease in diarrhea-associated but not other mortality in this period, has led to the conclusion that the program efforts resulted in the mortality reduction. However, because there were other changes during this time period, such as improvement in immunization coverage, changes in nutritional status, and enhancement of other health services, the direct contribution of the diarrheal disease control program or of other health programs cannot be quantified with certainty.

Unfortunately, few studies of the mortality impact of ORT programs have been done in other areas, and none have been done in sub-Saharan Africa. A study in India provided oral rehydration solution at a community level for episodes of diarrhea and reached levels of usage of up to 68 percent in study areas (Kumar et al., 1987). This study reported a substantial decrease in case-fatality rates and about a 60 percent reduction in diarrhea-associated deaths. However, the total childhood mortality rate in the areas differed by less than 10 percent from the rate in control areas.

The available studies suggest that childhood mortality can be reduced by diarrheal case-management programs that achieve a level of coverage of approximately 50-60 percent and effective use of oral rehydration therapy for diarrheal episodes. However, national diarrheal disease control programs have been variable in their success in achieving high coverage and effective use of ORT. Globally, it is estimated that 36 percent of diarrheal episodes are treated with ORT and the rate of use in sub-Saharan Africa is estimated by WHO to be similar (Programme for Control of Diarrhoeal Diseases, 1991b). However, it is recognized that ORT is not always utilized correctly (Touchette et al., 1990). Figure 4-1 illustrates the use of ORT during recent episodes of diarrhea, based on data from eight Demographic and Health Surveys (DHS) conducted in sub-Saharan Africa. A wide range of 3 to 72 percent is observed. In some countries, such as Botswana, Burundi, and Ghana, commercially prepared oral rehydration salts (ORS) are used more frequently. In Kenya and Nigeria, home-prepared solutions are used more often. (Zimbabwe did not report data on ORS.) Although approximately 70 percent of recent childhood diarrheal episodes received ORT according to the DHS in Botswana and Kenya, only 19 and 29 percent, respectively, of these cases were said to have received more fluids, as they should have (Boerma et al., 1991). Furthermore, although the recommendation is to continue the use of solid foods as before the illness, approximately half of the children in both of these settings were said to have been given less solid food during their illness. Also, the use of drugs, most of them unnecessary and some hazardous, remains quite high.

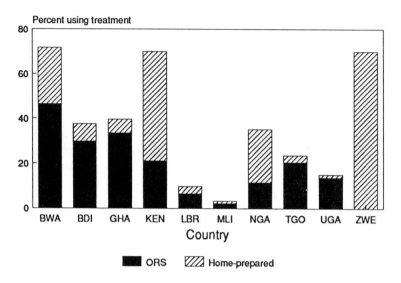

FIGURE 4-1 Use of oral rehydration therapy among children under 5 years of age, selected countries of sub-Saharan Africa. NOTE: Cases of diarrhea reported in the two weeks prior to survey. BWA—Botswana, BDI—Burundi, GHA—Ghana, KEN-Kenya, LBR—Liberia, MLI—Mali, NGA—Nigeria, TGO—Togo, UGA—Uganda, ZWE—Zimbabwe. SOURCE: Demographic and Health Survey reports (see Appendix B).

In eight DHS that collected information on the use of drugs during recent episodes of diarrhea, the median value was approximately 30 percent of episodes having received drugs, with a range of 10 to 44 percent (Boerma et al., 1990).

Demographic and Health Surveys can also be used to examine differentials in the use of ORT for treatment of diarrhea. Although children in the first six months of life may have a high risk of dehydration and subsequent mortality when they have diarrhea, eight DHS in sub-Saharan Africa (Botswana, Burundi, Ghana, Kenya, Liberia, Mali, Togo, and Uganda) consistently found that this age group had the lowest rate of use of ORT for diarrhea. In these surveys, there is evidence that use of ORS packets was higher in urban than in rural areas, with the exception of Kenya. In all countries except Uganda, there were higher rates of use of ORS among mothers with more education. ORS use was also higher in all countries in households with a radio. Thus, appropriate case management of diarrhea may still be inadequate in reaching the socially and economically disadvantaged populations of these countries, populations that are likely to have higher rates of childhood mortality.

With the severe limitations of data from sub-Saharan Africa, it is almost impossible to make calculations of current or future reductions in child mortality because of diarrheal disease control program efforts. However, even simplistic calculations can provide a perspective on the relative magnitude of the mortality impact that might be expected. For illustrative purposes, we assume that (1) 50 percent of diarrhea-associated mortality can be prevented by ORT if it is used optimally, and (2) currently 35 percent of diarrheal episodes are treated in the countries of sub-Saharan Africa, but (3) only 50 percent of these are treated effectively. Given these assumptions, we can calculate the maximum effect on diarrhea-associated mortality by multiplying these fractions together. Thus, these calculations would suggest that present levels of diarrheal disease control program efforts in sub-Saharan Africa may be reducing diarrhea-associated mortality in children under 5 years of age by approximately 9 percent. If 40 percent of deaths under age 5 are associated with diarrhea, then these programs might be reducing mortality under age 5 by about 3 or 4 percent. Additional reduction of diarrhea-associated child mortality could be achieved by increasing the number of episodes treated with ORT, improving the quality of diarrheal management, and widening program focus to address more fully the problems of dysentery and persistent diarrhea.

SUMMARY

Diarrheal diseases are a major contributing cause of infant and child mortality worldwide. The median number of episodes among children under 5 in studies in sub-Saharan Africa was 4.9 per year, with peak rates occurring between ages 6 and 18 months. Estimates of mortality due to diarrhea vary widely across studies and across populations. However, diarrheal diseases are often among the top three causes of death.

Most interventions directed at diarrheal disease focus on the management of acute dehydrating diarrhea by using oral rehydration therapy and continued feeding. Little emphasis has been placed on antibiotic therapy for treating dysentery or on dietary management for persistent diarrhea. Oral rehydration therapy is commonly used, and both hospital-based and community-based studies show that it is efficacious in reducing mortality from dehydrating acute watery diarrhea, but may be of limited use for treating dysentery and persistent diarrhea. No evaluations of the mortality effect of ORT have been conducted in sub-Saharan Africa, and virtually all research conducted in the region has been hospital based. Although it is an effective treatment, it is often used incorrectly or not given to infants under 6 months of age.

There is a need for more research on how to improve the coverage and the quality of home-based treatment and on the mortality impact of programs that encourage the use of ORT. Research on educational and other programs could contribute to a reduced incidence of the infections that cause diarrhea. Because the effect might be a reduction in mortality under age 5 of less than 5 percent, it would be very difficult to design studies that could document the effect of the programs on mortality rates.

MALARIA CONTROL PROGRAMS

Malaria is one of the major causes of death in Africa, and it is almost certainly responsible for the largest number of healthy days of life lost to disease in the entire population of certain countries (Ghana Health Assessment Team, 1981). It accounts for 20 to 60 percent of all illness seen in health facilities in the region, even though a large proportion of cases are treated only at home (Campbell, 1991). The World Health Organization has estimated that there are 1 to 2 million deaths worldwide from malaria each year (World Health Organization Scientific Group on the Chemotherapy of Malaria, 1990); most of these are in sub-Saharan Africa. Malaria mortality and morbidity may actually be increasing (Greenberg et al., 1989; Brinkmann and Brinkmann, 1991) as malaria moves into areas where it was previously absent or under control (e.g., Trape, 1987; Gascon et al., 1988, quoted by Brinkmann and Brinkmann, 1991).

The treatment of malaria is increasingly complicated by resistance to chloroquine. Brinkmann and Brinkmann (1991) concluded that in most countries of Africa, chloroquine resistance is found in from 25 to more than 60 percent of children. Recent studies have documented chloroquine resistance in all areas of the continent including most recently Senegal (Trape et al., 1989), Liberia (Björkman et al., 1991), and other parts of West Africa (Moran and Bernard, 1989), Somalia (Warsame et al., 1991), and South Africa (Freese et al., 1991). However, treatment with chloroquine remains effective in the majority of cases.

EPIDEMIOLOGY

Malaria is a parasitic disease that is spread by mosquitoes. Various stages of the parasite's life cycle must take place inside mosquitoes, so direct transmission between individuals is not possible except through blood transfusion. Therefore, the study of malaria transmission and of potential control measures includes studies of the biology of the parasite, the life cycle of mosquitoes, and the natural history of the disease in man.

There are several species of malaria. The most dangerous species is *Plasmodium falciparum*, which is very common in Africa. Other types include *P. vivax*, *P. ovale*, and *P. malariae*. The clinical manifestations of malaria often include a cycle of shaking chills, intense fevers, and drenching sweats. However, the symptoms vary greatly, especially among individuals who have acquired some immunity to the disease. Severe cases, generally from *P. falciparum*, can lead rapidly to death, often from cerebral malaria—a type of malaria in which the parasites clog capillaries in the brain. Other severe complications include renal failure, hypoglycemia, severe anemia, pulmonary edema, and shock. The wide range of symptoms can make diagnosis difficult. A definitive diagnosis of malaria infection is based on microscopic verification of the presence of parasites in the blood.

The epidemiology of malaria depends on the environment and its effect on the mosquito population. Malarious areas have been characterized by the level and seasonality of transmission as holoendemic (if transmission is year-round), hyperendemic (seasonal transmission), mesoendemic (a low level of transmission with occasional severe epidemics), or hypoendemic (limited transmission).

Individuals who have had repeated cases of malaria can develop partial immunity to it. However, repeated exposure is required to maintain this immunity. Thus, adults in holoendemic areas often have high levels of immunity. In mesoendemic regions, transmission is not frequent enough to maintain high levels of immunity. Thus, the severity of malarial infections is related to the level of transmission. Because children must have malaria before they can develop effective levels of immunity, malaria mortality is especially high in children in holoendemic and hyperendemic areas.

The Institute of Medicine Committee on Malaria Prevention and Control (Oakes et al., 1991) recently completed a report that covered a wide range of issues, including the current state of knowledge about the disease, the efficacy of current drugs, the economics of malaria, and priorities for research on new drugs and vaccines. The report presented eight paradigms that describe the range of ecologies in which malaria persists. These paradigms are not a complete classification system; they merely suggest the variety of circumstances in which malaria presents a serious health problem.

The paradigm that characterizes most of the areas in Africa where malaria is a serious health problem is the African savanna. The report (Oakes et al., 1991:217-218) states that

> eighty percent of the world's malaria and 90 percent of mortality due to the disease occur in Africa south of the Sahara, mostly in the savannah regions . . . . Malaria transmission is seasonal and correlates with relatively predictable patterns of rainfall, although transmission may continue at lower levels during the dry season. Because of the extremely high inoculation rates, virtually all of those living in these areas become infected early in life. For children, treatment . . . may prevent death long enough for acquired immunity to establish itself, which can provide protection from malaria-related death or illness later in life. Young children who do not

acquire this protective immunity, and whose infections are not treated adequately or promptly, are at particular risk of dying from the disease.

Six of the other seven paradigms are also represented in parts of Africa:

1. forest malaria, which describes parts of equatorial and central Africa;
2. malaria associated with irrigated agriculture, including the commercial cotton farms of the Gezira in the Sudan;
3. highland fringe malaria, in parts of Ethiopia and the mountain slopes of Kenya;
4. desert fringe and oasis malaria, found in areas such as the Sahel, on the fringes of the Kalahari desert, and in parts of Ethiopia;
5. urban malaria; and
6. seashore malaria.[1]

In some areas, the features of the environment and the disease suggest a combination of these paradigms, such as riverine malaria, which "is usually an intensification of either plains malaria or African savannah malaria, and associated with greater potential for vector breeding" (Oakes et al., 1991:221).

The diversity of malaria in sub-Saharan Africa is so great that there is no consensus on the best ways to approach the disease. There is agreement that no single approach makes sense for all types of areas (Oakes et al., 1991). However, national health programs have very limited resources for evaluating the situation in each local area.

MALARIA MORTALITY IN SUB-SAHARAN AFRICA

Estimates of mortality and morbidity from malaria are uncertain even in the best of circumstances. For example, in an excellent study of malaria mortality in The Gambia, 23 of 25 children who died of malaria died at home, 2 died in a dispensary, and none died in the hospital. Only six had received any treatment for the final illness other than traditional medicine or treatment at home (Greenwood et al., 1987). Therefore, few of these cases were ever seen by modern health workers and most of the deaths were ascribed to malaria using verbal autopsies.

In many studies, diagnosis of cause of death is based on information collected in verbal autopsies, although diagnosis is uncertain even in a clinical setting (Bassett et al., 1991). Simple microscopic tests can improve diagnosis. However, even when performed correctly this approach is prob-

---

[1] They also describe plains malaria associated with traditional agriculture, which is most common in South Asia and Central America.

lematic. In nonimmune patients, symptoms can arise from very low rates of parasitemia (i.e., parasites in the blood), which may become apparent only after repeated blood films. Moreover, when parasites are detected, there is no way to establish that the malaria infection is responsible for the observed symptoms. This lack of clarity is especially common for individuals with partial immunity to the disease who may be asymptomatic when infected (Oakes et al., 1991).

Good estimates of the contribution of malaria to child mortality rates in Africa are currently not available. The studies of causes of death reviewed in Chapter 2 suggest that malaria is often the third or fourth leading cause of mortality under age 5. However, the sensitivities and specificities of the usual criteria for diagnosing malaria by verbal autopsies are not very high. Therefore, estimates from verbal autopsies are probably useful only in age groups or seasons where malaria is responsible for 10 to 25 percent of deaths.

Greenwood et al. (1987) estimated that in a rural area of The Gambia, the malaria mortality rate was 6.3 per 1,000 among infants and 10.7 among children aged 1-4 years. These rates amounted to 4 percent of infant deaths and 25 percent of child deaths. However, it is likely that malaria mortality rates in this area vary substantially from year to year. A study of children less than 3 years of age in a coastal area of Benin estimated that the death rate due to malaria was probably about 8 deaths per 1,000 children (95 percent confidence interval (C.I.) 3.7-14.2 deaths per 1,000 children) (Velema et al., 1991). The rate was highest in the second year of life (14.9 per 1,000 children, 95 percent C.I. 11.2-18.6 per 1,000 children). A hospital-based study in Kinshasa, Zaire, estimated that the mortality rate to malaria was at least 4 per 1,000 in infants and 1.6 per 1,000 at ages 1-4 years (Greenberg et al., 1989).

PROGRAM OPTIONS

In 1959, the Eighth World Health Assembly adopted the goal of eradicating malaria. However, sub-Saharan Africa was excluded from immediate plans for eradication because of the perceived magnitude of the malaria problem and the lack of technical and organizational capability in the region. There were success stories during the 1950s and 1960s, especially in cities and at higher altitudes (e.g., Taylor and Mutambu, 1986). However, the goal of eradication proved to be elusive. In 1960, the World Health Assembly revised its global malaria strategy to emphasize control of malaria in areas where eradication was not possible.

The complex epidemiology of malaria provides several stages at which interventions can reduce the transmission or severity of cases. Spraying with insecticides and eliminating mosquito breeding grounds reduce the population of mosquitoes. If the number of mosquitoes is reduced enough, malaria incidence rates will fall. Bed nets and mosquito coils can reduce the incidence of mosquito bites and thereby reduce transmission from mosquitoes to humans. Chemoprophylaxis is the use of antimalarial drugs (often chloroquine or mefloquine) to protect against malarial infections. Treatment of cases (or presumed cases) of malaria reduces the severity and duration of the disease.

During the 1950s, most antimalarial programs were based on spraying with insecticides. This approach requires regular coverage to all areas for extended periods of time. It also requires careful monitoring of the levels of insecticide resistance among mosquitoes or the introduction of progressively more expensive insecticides. In most parts of Africa, these malarial control programs have not been sustainable because of the high degree of organization required and the increasing costs associated with insecticide resistance. However, some of the best evidence on the potential effects of malaria control on mortality comes from research on the effect of spraying programs.

The following sections review the evidence of the effect of malaria eradication on mortality and the effectiveness of three types of antimalarial programs. The first is presumptive treatment of suspected cases with antimalarial drugs, which includes both a review of the effect of programs designed to increase the proportion of cases treated with chloroquine and a review of studies of the importance of self-treatment. The second is chemoprophylaxis for pregnant women, which is designed to reduce the incidence of complications of pregnancy, low birthweight, and anemia among children. Finally, we briefly examine the potential of bed nets treated with insecticide.

Today the outlook for global eradication of malaria is very dim. The spread of drug-resistant malaria and insecticide-resistant mosquitoes has made control even more difficult than it was 20 years ago. One promising change is the development of malaria vaccines. There is evidence that immunization with various antigens can both reduce the consequences of malaria infections and help to disrupt transmission of the disease. However, efficacious vaccines will not be available for large-scale use for several years (Oakes et al., 1991).

STUDIES OF THE EFFECT OF MALARIA ERADICATION ON MORTALITY

There have been three studies attempting to eradicate malaria from small areas of Africa. These studies suggest the importance of malaria, but do not offer practical solutions for reducing its effect.

Pare-Taveta Malaria Scheme (1954-1959)

Conducted in northeastern Tanzania, the Pare-Taveta project reduced malaria transmission to very low levels through residual spraying of houses with dieldrin. The crude death rate dropped from about 24 per 1,000 to between 12 and 16 per 1,000 of all ages following spraying, and the infant mortality rate dropped from a range of 165-260 per 1,000 live births to between 78 and 132 deaths per 1,000 live births (Draper, 1962; Bradley, 1991a).

A second study, the Pare-Taveta Vital Statistics Survey (Pringle and Matola, 1967), covered the period 1962 to 1966 after the spraying program ended. It was designed to determine whether mortality returned to previous high levels. Although mortality at ages 1-4 returned to the earlier levels, mortality at other ages remained at the new lower levels. There were extensive investigations into the entomological and parasite biology and ecology to try to explain this result. The researchers concluded that the lower mortality rates were sustained in most age groups by a substantial, though undocumented, increase in the use of antimalarial drugs for presumptive treatment of fevers (Draper et al., 1972; Bradley, 1991a).

Kisumu Project

The Kisumu project tested the effect of residual spraying with fenitrothion on mortality in a district of Kenya (Payne et al., 1976). The daily malaria incidence rate dropped by about 96 percent in the program area. The crude death rate in the treated area declined from 24 deaths per 1,000 in the year preceding the spraying to 16 and 13.5 during the two subsequent years. The death rate in the control area actually increased slightly from 23 to 26 and 24, respectively, in the two subsequent years. The infant mortality rate dropped from 157 deaths per 1,000 in unprotected infants to 93—a 41 percent reduction. The drop in infant mortality affected only infants over 3 months of age.

Garki Project

The Garki project tested the effects of house spraying and prophylactic drug use on malaria in the northern part of Nigeria (Molineaux and Gramiccia, 1980). This area is part of the Sudan savanna that runs across Africa from Senegal to the Sudan. In the Garki area, transmission of malaria was more intense and more seasonal than in Kisumu (Molineaux, 1985). The project tested residual spraying with propoxur, both with and without periodic mass drug administration. In one area there was distribution of sulfalene-pyrimethamine every 10 weeks; in a second area, the frequency of distribution was increased to every 2 weeks during the wet seasons when malaria was most prevalent.

Before the start of the program, about 47 percent of the population tested positive for *Plasmodium falciparum* during the dry season and about 60 percent during the wet season (Molineaux and Gramiccia, 1980). Spraying alone brought about little change in the prevalence of infection. During the first wet season, prevalence in the spraying area was only 15 percent below the rate in the control area. During the second dry season, it was 26 percent below the rate in the control area. House spraying was not as successful in Garki as it was in Kisumu because a large proportion of the mosquitoes in Garki remained outside the houses and were not affected by spraying. During the dry season, the addition of mass drug administration every 10 weeks dropped the prevalence to 98 percent below the rate in the control area, but did not interrupt transmission. In the second wet season, the prevalence was only 72 percent below the rate in the control area. More frequent drug distribution reduced the prevalence by at least 95 percent, but still did not interrupt transmission.

The demographic data collected by the Garki project were extensive. However, the analysis of the data was weak and the sample size was small, leaving a number of questions unanswered. The mortality data for the baseline year suggested that it was not typical. The infant mortality rate (IMR) during the baseline was 246 deaths per 1,000 live births. During the following two years the IMR in the control area was only 155.[2] This difference is significant at the 5 percent level.[3] During the first intervention year, the IMR was 135 in the control area and only 55 in the treatment area (all treatments combined). For the whole intervention period the rates were 155 and 73, which are significantly different at the 5 percent level. However, we do not know how much of this difference between the control area and the intervention areas might be due to differences that existed before the start of the program. Although Molineaux and Gramiccia (1980) reported that the IMRs in the intervention and control areas were not significantly different at the baseline, they do not report the actual values. They also did not present the IMRs separately for the spraying area and the area that received both spraying and mass drug administration. The data in the figures showing seasonal fluctuations suggest that the decline in the IMR was larger in both types of intervention areas than in the control area (Molineaux

---

[2] This estimation combines nine deaths in the first intervention year with the seven deaths occurring during the period through the wet season (Molineaux and Gramiccia, 1980:237) among infants.

[3] The significance test compared the estimates of the age-specific mortality rate at age zero (i.e., $_1M_0$), which were used to estimate the IMR. For the sample size, we used the number of person-years of observation.

and Gramiccia, 1980:237-239, Figures 68-70). However, without baseline data for the various areas, we do not know if the differences between the declines were statistically significant.

The link between malaria control and differences in the IMR in the intervention and control areas was strengthened by the relationship between the infant death rates and the infant parasitological conversions rate (ICR), which measured the rate at which infants became infected. During the baseline year and in the control area data, there was a close relationship between the seasonal patterns of the IMR and the ICR. With the start of the program, the seasonal pattern disappeared and the IMR dropped in the intervention areas.

The mortality rate at 1-4 years also appears to have dropped in both the control and the intervention areas during the first year of intervention. However, the decrease in the areas that received both insecticide and mass drug administration (70 percent) was much larger than the drop in the control area and the area that received only insecticide (both about 25-30 percent). There was also a sharp change in the seasonal pattern of mortality in the intervention area. Molineaux and Gramiccia (1980) did not present an analysis of changes in mortality over age 5.

The Garki project demonstrated that in some environments in Africa it is not feasible to interrupt transmission of malaria. Even with extensive spraying and frequent distribution of prophylactic drugs, the Garki project never interrupted transmission even during the dry seasons. The high cost of this intensive approach and the complications introduced by insecticide and drug resistance reinforce this conclusion.

PRESUMPTIVE TREATMENT OF FEVERS WITH ANTIMALARIAL DRUGS

Each of the three projects reviewed above demonstrated that mortality under age 5 would decline if we could greatly reduce or eliminate malaria. However, there is currently no feasible method for accomplishing these tasks in most of Africa. The high costs and the heavy logistical requirements of control programs are among the reasons for this conclusion. Also supporting this conclusion are the exceedingly high transmission rates of malaria in much of Africa. In some areas, rates are so high that a program would have to reduce transmission by a factor of as much as a thousand to bring malaria under control (Bradley, 1991b). Therefore, as Campbell (1991:1,208) has noted "the challenge for control of malaria in African children is to develop operational strategies that will minimize the risks of illness without eliminating the continued exposure to infection necessary for maintaining clinical immunity."

Aggressive programs to provide chemotherapy are often advocated to achieve this balance. In most cases these programs take the form of presumptive treatment with chloroquine of all childhood fevers in malarious areas during malaria seasons. The practical reason for presumptive treatment of all fevers is that in areas where malaria is a serious problem, it is not feasible to identify those fevers that are due to malaria, even when microscopy is available and performed correctly (Bradley, 1991b; Oakes et al., 1991). Moreover, in most of Africa, microscopic verification is not available.

The potential efficacy of presumptive treatment depends in part on the proportion of fever cases that are attributable to malaria. Greenwood et al. (1987) estimated that in a rural area of The Gambia, only 40 percent of cases of fever in children under age 7 were attributable to malaria. In a monthly household survey in Benin, only about 33 percent of fever cases in children under 3 years of age were attributed to malaria (Velema et al., 1991).

Even if the fever is not caused by malaria, treating a preexisting case of malaria may reduce the overall infectious load enough to increase the child's chance of surviving. For example, Greenwood et al. (1987) found that 64 percent of fever cases had malaria parasites in their blood. The proportion of fever attributable to malaria, and therefore the potential of presumptive treatment, vary across areas and often by season. At a health clinic in Niamey, Niger, 54 percent of children with fever in the rainy season had malaria. However, in the dry season, only 3.6 percent had malaria (Olivar et al., 1991). Thus, these proportions may understate the potential for presumptive treatment.

There are many questions about the long-term efficacy of presumptive therapy in reducing mortality in Africa. In some cases, presumptive treatment may simply delay the onset of a massive attack. For example, such a delay has been suggested as an explanation for the appearance of cerebral malaria in teenagers in Banjul, The Gambia (Bradley, 1991b).

Chloroquine is still the most commonly used drug for presumptive treatment because of its safety and low cost. However, the efficacy of chloroquine is reduced in much of the continent by chloroquine resistance. As chloroquine resistance increases, many cases still show clinical improvement immediately following treatment (e.g., reduced fever). However, fever and other symptoms can return very quickly because of a failure to completely clear all parasites. When treatment fails within a few weeks, the child may not be able to recover fully from the attack. A study in Malawi (Centers for Disease Control, 1991) demonstrated that anemic children with malaria did not recover from the anemia after treatment with chloroquine. However, those treated with Fansidar showed increased hemoglobin levels within three weeks. Chloroquine resistance may be the cause of the reported increasing severity of pediatric anemia (Greenberg et al., 1989).

Studies of the Effect of Programs Designed to Increase Presumptive Treatment of Fevers with Chloroquine

Three basic strategies can be used to increase the proportion of fever cases treated with antimalarial drugs. The first is to encourage parents to take children to a health center whenever they have fever. A second is to train village health workers to treat fevers with antimalarials and to refer serious cases to a health center. The third strategy is to encourage home use of antimalarials for treatment of simple cases of fever. There are two studies conducted in Kenya and The Gambia that examine the efficacy of programs that rely on village health workers to treat cases of fever with chloroquine, as well as one study of an education program to increase home use.

Saradidi Health Development Project

The Saradidi Health Development Project was a community health program in western Kenya based on village-level organizations and "village health helpers" (VHHs) (Kaseje and Sempebwa, 1989). The program raised funds to build buildings for clinics, maternity services, and other facilities necessary for providing community health services. The VHHs provided health education on topics including environmental health, promotion of maternal and child health services and immunizations, family planning, and nutrition education. In selected areas, they provided antimalarial chemoprophylaxis (i.e., use of drugs to prevent infection) for pregnant women and treatment for malaria. A comparison of mortality rates before and during the community-based malaria control intervention showed a significant decline in child mortality (ages 1-4 years) in the intervention areas (from 25.5 to 18.2 per 1,000). However, this decline was apparently due to lower measles mortality and not to the antimalarial activities (Spencer et al., 1987). The research team concluded that "the most likely reason for the lack of any detectable effect is that there was already a high level of chloroquine use for illness presumed to be due to malaria before the program" (Spencer et al., 1987:14). The main change in treatment patterns was a change in the source of chloroquine from shops and health clinics to the village health helpers (Mburu et al., 1987).

Village Health Workers in The Gambia

A study in The Gambia (Greenwood et al., 1988; Menon et al., 1990) compared mortality and malaria morbidity rates in three areas. Two areas were included in the government's primary health care (PHC) program. In both areas, village health workers (VHWs) learned to treat malaria with chloroquine. In one of the areas the VHWs also distributed, every two weeks, malaria chemoprophylaxis or a placebo to all children aged 3-59 months of age. Children were allocated to the chemoprophylaxis or placebo group randomly by compound. The third area was not covered by the PHC program, but treatment of malaria was available from a dispensary.

The authors (Greenwood et al., 1988:1,125) summarized their results for 9 to 21 months after the start of the program as follows:

> Treatment of presumptive clinical malaria by VHWs with chloroquine had no significant effect on mortality and morbidity from malaria in young Gambian children whilst treatment combined with malaria chemoprophylaxis given by VHWs reduced mortality and morbidity in children aged 1-4 years . . . . [C]hemoprophylaxis did not reduce mortality in infants aged 3-11 months, for . . . malaria accounts for only about 4% of deaths in infants.

The results remained the same in a second study 33 to 45 months after the start of the program (Menon et al., 1990).

For whatever reasons, the program apparently did not lead to a large increase in presumptive treatment of fevers with chloroquine. Because the VHWs were only voluntary workers, they may not have been able to provide sufficient coverage for acute episodes. In the villages with primary health care, children received an average of 0.52 regimens of chloroquine per year, which included an average of 0.34 regimens distributed by the VHWs and 0.18 regimens from a dispensary. In the non-PHC villages, children received an average of 0.42 regimens from a dispensary. Both averages are probably too low in a community where children have an average of 0.5 to 1.0 clinical episode of malaria per year. Therefore, the VHWs failed to achieve a meaningful increase in the proportion of cases treated with chloroquine. However, the study did not provide information on whether the use of VHWs changed the promptness of treatment, amount of drug taken, or duration of treatment.

Conclusions About the Effectiveness of Programs to Increase Presumptive Treatment

Because the village workers in both of these programs failed to increase treatment levels significantly, the studies do not provide tests of the efficacy of presumptive treatment. Instead they test the use of village health workers to increase presumptive treatment. Therefore, we still do not know what would happen if we could achieve presumptive treatment of all fevers with chloroquine.

It may not be possible to conduct a trial of presumptive treatment with chloroquine because in most places where malaria is a significant problem, presumptive treatment of fevers is already common. Case-control studies would be hindered by problems of retrospective reporting of general treatment practices as well as specification errors resulting from use of other modern treatments for other diseases. It may be that studies could be based on prospective surveys comparing families that report relying on use of chloroquine with other families. However, even this approach is not likely to provide a reliable estimate of the efficacy of presumptive treatment because of the likelihood of other differences between these two groups of families.

Studies of Self-Treatment

Self-treatment of fevers with antimalarials (generally chloroquine) is very common in many parts of sub-Saharan Africa. The term self-treatment refers to treatment that was not given during or after a visit to a health center. It can include, but is not limited to, use that was recommended by a pharmacy, commercial shop, or traditional healer. In general, self-treatment is based on drugs acquired at a shop or from a health clinic during a visit for a previous disease episode. Table 4-1 summarizes the importance of self-treatment found in studies in eight areas of Africa. Between 8 and 98 percent of children received self-treatment for fevers.

Data from the Demographic and Health Surveys suggest that self-treatment is very common. Most of the DHS in Africa inquired about recent cases of fever among children 1-59 months of age. They generally asked whether the child was taken to a medical facility and what treatments were received. Table 4-2 shows that antimalarial use was reported for 20 to 74 percent of recent cases of fever among children and that in most of the surveys, about half of the recent cases of fever were treated at a medical facility (Burundi, Ghana, Kenya, Senegal, and Uganda all reported values between 48 and 58 percent). In Botswana, 90 percent reported going to a medical facility, whereas 3 percent did in Mali and 31 percent in Togo.

The DHS did not ask where the drugs were acquired or whether they were prescribed by a doctor. Therefore, we do not know how many children received antimalarials before going to a clinic. However, we can derive a minimum estimate by looking at the proportion of children who reportedly received antimalarials but did not attend a health facility. Table 4-2 shows that in the five countries where the DHS provides the relevant information, 9 to 35 percent of recent cases of fever among children were reportedly treated by antimalarials but not at a health facility. It is likely that many children who did attend a clinic received antimalarials before going to the clinic. This is especially true for Ghana, Senegal, and Uganda, where about half of all children with fever were taken to a health clinic.

The most detailed study of self-treatment of fever was carried out by Deming et al. (1989) in the Plateaux Region of Togo. They found that 83

TABLE 4-1 Home-Based Presumptive Treatment of
Fevers in Children with Antimalarial Drugs, Eight
Areas of Sub-Saharan Africa

Area	Cases of Fever Receiving Antimalarials at Home (%)
Urban	
Ghana (Accra)	56
Guinea (Conakry)	51
Rural	
Ghana (Berekuso)	98
Guinea (Dinguiraye)	13
Guinea (Dabola)	21
Rwanda (national)	8
Togo (Plateaux)	83
Zaire (Kingandu and Pai-Kongila)	28

NOTE: Estimates for Ghana assume that the distribution of drugs
used for treating fever is the same for home treatment (which accounted for 87 and 94 percent, respectively, of treatments) as for all
treatment.

SOURCE: Deming (1989), except for data from Ghana, which is from
Gardiner et al. (1984).

percent of children with a recent case of suspected fever were treated with
antimalarial drugs (almost always chloroquine) at home before attending or
instead of attending a clinic. Mothers stated that virtually all (97 percent)
children treated at home with antimalarials began treatment on the first day
of their fever. In contrast, only 17 percent of children who were taken to a
clinic were taken on the first day of fever. This difference is of consequence, given the importance of early treatment (World Health Organization, 1990).

Deming et al. also compared the dose reported by mothers to that required for the child's weight. This comparison led to an estimated mean
dosage of 8.9 milligrams of chloroquine per kilogram of body weight during the first 24 hours of therapy. At the time of the survey, the recommended treatment with chloroquine was a single dose of 10 milligrams per
kilogram during the first 24 hours. The mean dosage did not differ significantly for children 0-1 and 2-4 years. Only 1 percent of reported dosages
during the first 24 hours were 20 milligrams per kilogram or higher, a value
taken to represent potentially serious toxicity. The mean total dose per
episode of malaria was 16.6 milligrams per kilogram.

It appears, therefore, that in at least one area of Africa, self-treatment
of presumed fever was very prompt and the reported dosages were very

TABLE 4-2 Treatment Patterns (percent) Among Children Aged 1-59 Months Who Had a Fever, Nine Countries of Sub-Saharan Africa

Country	Treated with Antimalarials	Taken to Health Center or Doctor	Treated with Antimalarials but did not Attend Health Center
Botswana	n.a.	90.2	n.a.
Burundi	19.8	49.9	8.8
Ghana	24.9	56.4	12.3
Kenya	n.a.	55.5	n.a.
Liberia	73.5	n.a.	n.a.
Mali	35.5	2.9	34.6
Senegal	26.7	57.6	17.9
Togo	56.5	30.8	n.a.
Uganda	57.1	48.3	28.0

NOTE: n.a. = not available.

SOURCE: Demographic and Health Survey reports (see Appendix B).

close to the recommended levels.[4] This result was obtained despite the fact that self-treatment was not promoted as a national policy or encouraged as an alternative to treatment at health centers, although it was recommended in local health education projects.

A study in The Gambia (Menon et al., 1988) tested an education program designed to improve self-treatment of malaria. In this area, they found that women knew little about the causes of malaria, and few (2 percent) reported that they would use chloroquine first if they thought their child had malaria. After an education campaign, 91 percent knew the correct treatment for various hypothetically ill children. In a prospective survey, about 70 percent of women gave chloroquine as instructed for treatment of fever. However, many also gave chloroquine for upper respiratory, gastrointestinal, and dermatological symptoms presumably not related to malaria.

This study suggests the potential for education programs aimed at proper treatment of fevers. However, it demonstrates that these education programs must be designed to help mothers identify malaria and to recognize serious cases that require immediate medical attention. This type of education program might be combined with a program that uses village health workers who could periodically reinforce the education messages.

---

[4]The recommended dosage in Togo were later changed to 25 milligrams per kilogram given over three days.

As noted earlier, self-treatment is not inconsistent with attendance at a health clinic. In a pilot study in Accra, Ghana (Orofi-Adjei et al., 1984), nine children presenting with fever and anemia were tested for serum chloroquine levels. Although only two cases admitted to using chloroquine prior to admission, seven of the children had chloroquine in their serum. Prior medication can complicate treatment at the clinic since prescription of additional chloroquine can lead to overdosing (World Health Organization, 1990). Also, continued treatment with chloroquine may unnecessarily delay treatment with other drugs in cases of chloroquine resistance.

PROGRAMS BASED ON CHEMOPROPHYLAXIS AMONG PREGNANT WOMEN

Chemoprophylaxis is the use of antimalarial drugs to prevent cases of malaria. The World Health Organization Scientific Group on the Chemotherapy of Malaria (1990) concluded that "chemoprophylaxis is only recommended at present for special risk groups, notably pregnant women, nonimmune travellers, and nonimmune persons living in closed communities in endemic areas for fixed predetermined periods (e.g., labor forces and police and army units)." For this reason, chemoprophylaxis is rarely a component of health programs in Africa. Therefore, we have not reviewed the extensive literature on the efficacy of chemoprophylaxis for young children. We have reviewed studies about use of chemoprophylaxis among pregnant women, which is a part of many health programs.

The recommendation of chemoprophylaxis during pregnancy rests on the following chain of reasoning:

Proposition 1: Malaria during pregnancy has been associated with anemia, miscarriage, fetal death, intrauterine growth retardation, low birthweight, and preterm delivery. Most studies find that these effects are concentrated in first pregnancies (i.e., primigravidae). See, for example, studies of low birthweight and malaria (Gilles, 1969; McGregor, 1984).

Proposition 2: Chemoprophylaxis during pregnancy can prevent or effectively treat malaria and reduce the incidence of low birthweight and anemia during pregnancy. Figure 4-2 presents the estimates of the effect of prophylaxis on birthweight in first births from six randomized trials in Africa (Burkina Faso—Cot et al., 1992; Uganda—Hamilton et al., 1972; The Gambia—Greenwood et al., 1989; Imesi, Nigeria—Morley et al., 1964; Ibadan, Nigeria—Gilles et al., 1969; and Zaria, Nigeria—Fleming et al., 1986). The studies differ substantially in sample size, so the width of the bars in the figure is roughly proportional to the inverse of the variance of the estimate of effect. The two largest studies (Hamilton et al., 1972; Cot et al., 1992) found difference in birthweights among first births of about 80 grams

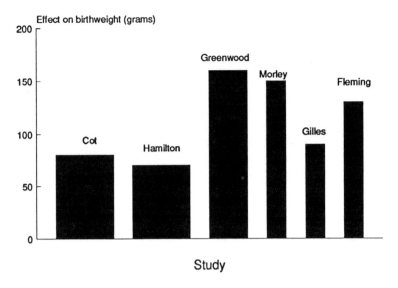

FIGURE 4-2 Effect of malaria prophylaxis on birthweight, first births in six randomized trials in Africa. NOTE: Width of bars proportional to the inverse of the variance of estimate. Sources: Morley et al. (1964); Gilles et al. (1969); Hamilton et al. (1972); Fleming et al. (1986); Greenwood et al. (1989); Cot et al. (1992).

associated with prophylaxis, although this difference was not significant in either study.[5] In the third largest trial (Greenwood et al., 1989), the estimated effect on first births was much greater and was significant at the 5 percent level. The overall average effect of prophylaxis in all of the studies was about 100 grams.[6] The similarity of the results is impressive, given the differences in study designs, treatment regimens, ecological settings, and levels of treatment provided to the control group. For example, the proportion of pediatric deaths in Togo ascribed to malaria or anemia increased steadily between 1986 and 1989 (Centers for Disease Control, 1991) and the number of cases of malaria reported in Burundi almost tripled between 1987 and 1992 (Republique du Burundi, 1993). In addition, case-fatality rates of malaria have increased in Zaire and the Central African Republic (Centers for Disease Control, 1991).

---

[5]For the study by Hamilton et al. (1972) the comparison is between women who received chloroquine and iron, and women who received only iron.

[6]Some of the studies have many more women in one group or the other (test or control). Therefore, we have averaged the estimates of the effect of prophylaxis, weighting each study by the geometric mean of the number of women in the two groups.

Four of the studies (Cot et al., 1992; Hamilton et al., 1972; Greenwood et al., 1989; Morley et al., 1964) give estimates for the effects in later pregnancies. These estimates are more difficult to compare because the studies grouped the parities differently and the largest study (Cot et al., 1992) did not provide a separate estimate for higher parity women.[7] It appears that prophylaxis has little or no effect on births of order 2 through 4, but may be beneficial among higher parity women.

Several of these studies also examined the effect of chemoprophylaxis on the incidence of anemia during pregnancy. Greenwood et al. (1989) found that prophylaxis affected hemoglobin levels only in the primigravidae. Gilles et al. (1969) and Fleming et al. (1986) also demonstrated this effect in primigravidae.

Proposition 3: Low birthweight is associated with increased risk of infant death. The literature on this topic is reviewed in Chapter 5.

Although the research supports each of these propositions, only two studies have been uncovered that present data on the effect of chemoprophylaxis on child survival. Greenwood et al. (1989) show that the stillbirth and neonatal mortality rates were lower among first pregnancies for women who received Maloprim than for women who received a placebo. However, the rates were not significantly different. When neonatal mortality and still-births are combined, first pregnancies led to a bad outcome 8.1 percent of the time for those on prophylaxis and 15.4 percent of the time for those on placebo (relative risk of 0.53 times; 95 percent C.I. 0.20-1.37 times). Among later pregnancies there was virtually no difference associated with prophy-laxis (4.4 percent compared to 6.0 percent for the control group). Morley et al. (1964) found no difference in the combined stillbirth and neonatal mor-tality rate associated with prophylaxis for women of all parities.

There are several ways the logic that links these three propositions could prove misleading. First, if the effect of chemoprophylaxis on birthweight is very small, it might not lead to any noticeable difference in child sur-vival. Second, most of the studies present data on mean birthweights. However, the proportion with low birthweight is probably a better measure of the potential effect on child survival. Cot et al. (1992) reported that the relative risk of low birthweight among primigravidae was 0.88 for those on prophylaxis, compared to the controls, although this difference was not significant. Greenwood et al. (1989) reported that prophylaxis was associ-

---

[7]Cot et al. (1992) showed that for women of all parities, the group that received prophylaxis had a mean birthweight only 5.6 grams higher than the control group. Since the difference for primigravidae was 82 grams, the multiparous in the prophylaxis group must have had a mean birthweight about 20 grams lower than the control group.

ated with a drop in the proportion with low birthweight among primigravidae from 22 to 5 percent (probability less than .05).

Third, some studies show that the rate of malaria parasitemia may decrease during the last trimester even without treatment (McGregor, 1984). If the growth retardation associated with malaria occurs at a different stage of pregnancy than retardation caused by other factors, the relationship between low birthweight and child survival may differ as well. Similarly, it is not clear whether malarial infections lead to short gestation or to growth retardation (i.e., low weight for gestational age).

Fourth, the use of chemoprophylaxis in pregnant women is complicated by the increasing prevalence of chloroquine resistance. Chloroquine is inexpensive, relatively safe, and well-tolerated, and the general policy on chemoprophylaxis during pregnancy relies heavily on these features of the drug. Although chloroquine may be more effective in adults who have partial immunity than in children, several studies have indicated high failure rates (i.e., breakthrough with a clinical attack of malaria during pregnancy) of chloroquine prophylaxis among pregnant women (McDermott et al., 1988; Mutabingwa et al., 1991). The alternatives to chloroquine for chemotherapy are quite limited. The Institute of Medicine (Oakes et al., 1991:67) concluded that "the safety and efficacy of alternative prophylactic regimens in pregnancy is an open question."

A study in Tanzania suggested that chloroquine is still a useful drug for pregnant women in areas where chloroquine resistance is common. However, chemoprophylaxis with a weekly dose of chloroquine was more apt to lead to failure than daily doses of proguanil (Mutabingwa et al., 1991).

McDermott et al. (1988) studied the efficacy of chloroquine in Malawi, which had had documented chloroquine resistance for several years. They found that chloroquine was successful in clearing malaria parasitemia in 9 of 19 pregnant women and may have reduced placental infection rates.[8] However, 25 percent of women (18 of 73) experienced breakthrough parasitemia during pregnancy while they were taking either chloroquine or amodiaquin, with no significant difference between the two drugs.

Finally, programs designed to deliver prophylaxis to pregnant women would have to address the issue of coverage rates and compliance. For example, a study in Saradidi, Kenya, showed that only 29 percent of pregnant women attending maternal and child clinics were taking chemoprophylaxis, despite a program that used village health helpers to encourage its use. Only 25 percent of pregnant women aged 15-29 were taking chemoprophylaxis

---

[8]Breakthrough occurred in 2 of 36 women using chemoprophylaxis and in 7 of 36 controls (probability less than .10). The controls for this part of the study were women who had attended antenatal clinics and had access to unsupervised chloroquine chemoprophylaxis.

(Spencer et al., 1987). The World Health Organization Scientific Group on the Chemotherapy of Malaria (1990:80) has noted that in "well supervised studies . . . compliance [in children or adults] rarely exceeds 90% and generally ranges from 30% to 60%."

Heymann et al. (1990) addressed the issues of chloroquine efficacy and compliance in a study in Malawi. The program provided women at a prenatal clinic with a one-month supply of chloroquine. They estimated that chloroquine reduced the incidence of *Plasmodium falciparum* infection by only 23 percent among the 36 percent of pregnant women who complied. Therefore, the program prevented only about 8 percent of cases of infection among pregnant women.

It may be difficult to design studies that measure the effect of chemoprophylaxis on child survival. Because it has been determined that chemoprophylaxis increases birthweight, it may not be possible to withhold it for research purposes. Therefore, it might be necessary to rely on naturally occurring control areas or on evidence of changes in the level or seasonal pattern of infant mortality associated with increased prophylaxis. On the other hand, studies that directly address the question of child survival would have to overcome the problems of recording birthweights and gestational ages, both of which are very difficult to collect in Africa.

PROGRAMS BASED ON VECTOR CONTROL

Before the harmful effects of DDT and other residual insecticides were fully appreciated, considerable progress was achieved in the reduction of malaria mortality and morbidity through spraying. In some areas, mostly in cities and towns, these programs continue and are still effective in controlling the population of mosquitoes and malaria. More recently, greater stress has been laid on the use of personal protection against mosquito bites, including wearing long clothes, using mosquito coils, using ointments containing insecticide, and sleeping in mosquito nets (Rozendaal, 1989). None of these protective measures are part of a national strategy to control malaria, but more recently, the introduction of bed nets and curtains dipped in insecticide (permethrin is the most common) has been adopted as a community-based intervention against malaria in both adults and children. The experimental work on which these strategies are based took place in 1988-1990 in central Gambia, where Alonso and Greenwood showed that mortality in the test villages among children ages 1-4 was 37 percent below the rate in the control villages (Alonso et al., 1991). The trial also demonstrated that much of the decrease in mortality was due to the reduction of deaths identifiable as due to malaria by the verbal autopsy process (see Alonso et al., 1991; Greenwood and Pickering, 1993, for details).

The large reductions in malaria morbidity and mortality reported from the Gambian trial are unlikely to be repeated in national programs for various reasons associated with the capricious nature of the disease in relation to climatic and other ecological conditions, and to the difference between the effects anticipated in an experiment compared with those expected from a national program. Nonetheless, the use of treated bed nets seems worthy of further studies in other environments. One feature of the trial of impregnated bed nets is the larger than expected reduction in overall mortality. There are enormous problems in identifying a death due to malaria, but those aside, there seems to be some evidence in the changing cause-of-death distributions that other causes of death have also declined as a result of the reduction of malaria morbidity and mortality (see Alonso et al., 1991; Greenwood and Pickering, 1993, for a fuller discussion).

Several large trials of the effects of treated bed nets on malaria, childhood mortality and morbidity, and the birthweights of firstborn are in progress under the supervision of the World Health Organization (WHO). Apart from the problem of introducing bed nets into areas where they are uncommon, the principal obstacle to further use of the treated bed nets is the high recurring cost of the insecticide. Nonetheless, the evidence from the first year of the Gambian national intervention is very encouraging. There are measurable effects on the mosquito population, on the incidence of malaria illness, on childhood mortality, and on the birthweights of firstborn children (Cham and D'Alessandro, personal communication, 1992). Results from other national studies will soon be forthcoming.

SUMMARY

Malaria is a major cause of death and morbidity in Africa. There is substantial variation in the importance of malaria among various regions of sub-Saharan Africa, but in many populations it is the third or fourth most common cause of death. Studies in several areas have demonstrated that infant and child mortality could be reduced substantially if malaria were eliminated or greatly reduced. However, the design of antimalarial programs is complicated by the diversity of ecologies, the spread of chloroquine-resistant strains, and the high costs and managerial complexity of many of the available technologies.

Given the careful examination of strategies for malaria control by the World Health Organization (1984, 1990), the Institute of Medicine (Oakes et al., 1991), and the American Association for the Advancement of Science (1991), this report has not attempted a complete review of the evidence of the effectiveness of all approaches to reducing mortality to malaria. Rather, it has focused principally on three topics: use of village health workers to increase presumptive treatment of fevers, home-based presumptive treatment of fevers, and chemoprophylaxis during pregnancy.

Neither of the two major studies of the use of village health workers to increase presumptive treatment documented a reduction in child mortality. In both cases the programs failed to achieve an adequate increase in the proportion of cases treated. Therefore, we cannot conclude that an increase in presumptive treatment would not reduce child mortality.

These studies raise serious questions about the use of village health workers to increase presumptive treatment of fevers. We have not attempted a complete review of studies of coverage rates and compliance in programs of this sort. However, given the existing high rates of home-based use in many areas, the problems of managing and supplying large numbers of village health workers, the increasing prevalence of chloroquine resistance, and the lack of evidence of mortality reduction, it is not certain that programs based on village health workers can reduce child mortality by encouraging presumptive treatment.

It is still important for health clinics to provide presumptive treatment of fevers in areas and seasons during which malaria is a major cause of illness. The Institute of Medicine (IOM) identified this task as its first priority for malaria control (Oakes et al., 1991:16). In some areas where village health workers provide other services, adding presumptive treatment to their portfolios may be useful. The choice of appropriate drugs and treatment strategies must be worked out in each area, based on the prevalence of chloroquine resistance, the availability and affordability of alternatives, and the likelihood that patients will return to health clinics for further treatment if chloroquine fails.

It is well known that home-based treatment of fevers with chloroquine is very common in sub-Saharan Africa. However, there has been little research on self-treatment. Given the high frequency of this practice documented in numerous areas, there is a need for more studies of the drugs and dosages used, the promptness of self-treatment, and the ability of mothers to determine when it is important to take their children to a health center.

The paucity of data on self-treatment and the frequent emphasis on prevention rather than treatment have led most researchers to understate the potential importance of health education programs designed to encourage, discourage, or improve self-treatment. Efforts to increase the proper treatment of presumed cases of fever usually have been limited to treatment at health centers or by village health workers.

If self-treatment is found to be common and reasonably effective, then health education programs might focus on improving methods of recognizing symptoms of fevers, increasing knowledge of symptoms that require prompt modern treatment, and increasing awareness of the need for prompt treatment with appropriate dosages. If self-treatment is found to involve improper doses, to be used in inappropriate cases, or to delay or prevent seeking modern medical care in severe cases, then health education might discourage self-treatment and encourage prompt treatment at modern medical facilities. In either case, self-treatment is so prevalent that it cannot be ignored either as a potential opportunity to improve prompt presumptive treatment or as a hindrance to coverage of superior sources of treatment. In many populations, education programs designed to improve home-based presumptive treatment may be more cost-effective than programs based on village health workers. The potential effectiveness of self-treatment will also depend on the efficacy of chloroquine and the costs and perceived safety of alternative drugs that might be used for self-treatment.

Research on the effect of malaria control activities must involve monitoring of self-treatment and treatment at dispensaries. It is not adequate to consider an area as a pure "control" without consideration of existing treatment practices. For example, the Saradidi project in Kenya found that the main effect of the use of village health workers for treating presumptive cases of malaria was a change in the source of chloroquine. Similarly, the use of village health workers in The Gambia led to 57 percent less use of drugs from the dispensaries in the program area compared to the control, and only a 24 percent higher overall rate of treatment. Few of the large-scale studies of methods for preventing or treating malaria provide sufficient information about the baseline or control levels of prophylaxis or treatment.

The World Health Organization Scientific Group on the Chemotherapy of Malaria (1990) recommends chemoprophylaxis for pregnant women. However, the IOM committee and WHO Scientific Group on the Chemotherapy of Malaria both concluded that there is little evidence that prevention or reduction of malaria in pregnant women improves the prognosis for infants (World Health Organization Scientific Group on the Chemotherapy of Malaria 1990:85; Oakes et al., 1991:64-54, 234). There is strong evidence that chemoprophylaxis can increase mean birthweights among first births, but it is not clear to what extent this increase translates into higher child survival rates. No studies have examined the effect of chemoprophylaxis during pregnancy on the infant mortality rate, and there is little information about the effect on perinatal or neonatal mortality. In addition, there is little evidence from large-scale health programs. In these programs the effect of chemoprophylaxis is probably quite small, given that compliance is often low, not all women seek prenatal care early in their pregnancy, and the efficacy of chloroquine (the most commonly used drug) is declining in many areas.

ACUTE RESPIRATORY INFECTIONS

Acute respiratory infections (ARIs) are a group of upper and lower respiratory tract illnesses caused by bacterial, viral, or fungal infections. Of these infections, acute lower respiratory infections (ALRI), predominantly pneumonia, are the most serious and are major causes of mortality in developing countries among children under 5 years of age.

Studies in a number of developing countries, including The Gambia, Zaire, Nigeria, and Kenya, have indicated that serious and potentially fatal cases of pneumonia are predominantly due to two bacterial organisms *Streptococcus pneumoniae* and *Hemophilus influenzae*. This recognition and the success in individual cases of treatment with antibiotics have led to the predominance of a case management strategy for ARI control. This strategy is based on an algorithm that uses primarily respiratory rate and recognition of chest indrawing as a basis for diagnosis of pneumonia in children with cough, and on the appropriate treatment of such an illness with antibiotics (Programme for Control of Acute Respiratory Infections, 1990).

EPIDEMIOLOGY

The magnitude of the problem of acute respiratory infections in sub-Saharan Africa was reviewed recently by Kirkwood (1991), who summarized 42 studies from 21 countries (approximately half of the countries in this subregion). Whereas a number of studies reported on the high rates of all respiratory infections, few studies provided information on acute lower respiratory infections or pneumonia. A study in Kenya using both home and clinic surveillance found an incidence rate for ALRIs of 21 per 100 child-years (Selwyn, 1990). This rate is consistent with those found in other developing country settings, where the peak incidences appear to occur in the youngest children (Kirkwood, 1991).

In developing countries, pneumonia is thought to be one of the two most common causes of death in childhood. As summarized by Kirkwood (1991), studies that used an appropriate methodology to determine the cause-of-death structure among children under age 5 found that approximately 7.5 percent of these were due to pneumonia. Angola and Guinea-Bissau had age-specific mortality information available (Kirkwood, 1991). In these countries, the proportionate mortality from pneumonia was highest in children 1-4 years of age (15.2 percent in Angola and 8.9 percent in Guinea-Bissau). However, a larger number of deaths due to ARI occurred among infants because the infant mortality rates were substantially higher than the rates of children aged 1-4 years. The estimated mortality rates due to ARI globally are 10 to 30 deaths per 1,000 live births in infancy and 1.6 to 4.0 deaths per 1,000 children 1-4 years old (Foster, 1985).

There are a number of host and environmental risk factors for pneumonia in children. These include low birthweight, protein-energy malnutrition, lack of breastfeeding in young children, and possibly vitamin A deficiency. They also include exposure to air pollution, especially that caused by biomass fuel combustion in households. All of these factors would appear to be present in much of the sub-Saharan African population. Although it is not known to be a risk factor for pneumonia per se, malaria may complicate the diagnosis of pneumonia and the management of sick children.

A review of the sub-Saharan African DHS indicates that the incidence of ARI symptoms is greater among children living in rural areas than among those children living in urban areas. Little difference was observed in the incidence of ARI based on the mother's educational status.

INTERVENTIONS

A number of intervention trials have been initiated to test the effectiveness and feasibility of reducing pneumonia mortality through population-based case-management programs, which previously had not been attempted on a large scale. To date, results from seven intervention studies from around the world have been published and provide evidence for mortality reduction (Mtango and Neuvians, 1986; Datta et al., 1987; Pandey et al., 1989, 1991; Bang et al., 1990; Khan et al., 1990; Fauveau et al., 1992). A recent meta-analysis of the published case-management intervention trials provides a conservative estimate of an overall reduction of infant mortality by 15.9 deaths per 1,000 births and a cumulative under-5 mortality rate reduction of 36 deaths per 1,000 children (Sazawal and Black, 1992). These estimates would be consistent with a 20 percent reduction in infant mortality and a 25 percent reduction in all under-5 mortality for the studies analyzed.

The only one of these intervention trials in sub-Saharan Africa was in the Bagamoyo District of Tanzania (Mtango and Neuvians, 1986). In this study, episodes of pneumonia were sought by household visiting every six to eight weeks. In addition, women were taught about the need for seeking care if the child had certain signs and symptoms. All detected cases of pneumonia were treated with oral co-trimoxazole, and severe cases were referred to higher-level care. The difference in the mortality rate under age 5, $_5m_0$, was 7.7 deaths per 1,000 children (32.5 deaths per 1,000 children in the intervention area compared to 40.1 in the control area; 95 percent C.I. for difference was 2.0-13.5 deaths per 1,000 children). Thus, the probability of dying by age 5, $_5q_0$, was lower by 38.5 per 1,000 births, consistent with the meta-analysis of the other studies. The pneumonia-specific mortality rates declined by 30 percent over the two-year intervention period.

National efforts to implement the ARI case-management strategy have begun only in the last several years. As an indicator of performance, these programs use the proportion of pneumonia episodes needing antibiotics that actually receive them. In surveys, this indicator may be approximated by the proportion of recent cases of cough with rapid or difficult breathing that received antibiotics. Data from a few surveys conducted in sub-Saharan Africa are available on the current status of programs.

The data suggest a fairly consistent level of respiratory difficulties. In the Zimbabwe DHS, 7.6 percent of children 1-59 months of age had an episode of cough with rapid or difficult breathing in the four weeks preceding the survey (Boerma et al., 1991). In the Nigeria DHS, 6.7 percent reported to have had these symptoms sometime during the previous two weeks (Nigerian Federal Office of Statistics and Institute for Resource Development, 1992). In Mali and Togo, a question was asked about breathing problems of the children in the preceding two weeks (Boerma et al., 1991). The percentages of children with such a problem were 6.5 and 9.3, respectively.

In spite of these high levels, only a relatively small proportion receive medical attention in many countries. Of the children with respiratory difficulties in Mali, only 5.9 percent were taken to a medical facility, whereas in Togo, 33.2 percent were. On the other hand, in Kenya, 65 percent of children with respiratory complaints were taken to a medical facility. The proportion of children in these three countries treated appropriately with antibiotics could not be determined reliably from these surveys.

In Nigeria, mothers reported that 35 percent of these children with cough and rapid breathing were taken to a health facility or provider, 23 percent were given an antibiotic pill or syrup, and 23 percent received an unidentified injection (Nigerian Federal Office of Statistics and Institute for Resource Development, 1992). However, certain groups, such as children in rural areas and in families with lower levels of maternal education, were less likely to be taken to a medical facility. Thus, it is likely that the reduction in mortality will be proportionately lower in these groups than in other groups.

Even without an intensive ARI control program, existing medical services may be having some effect on reducing mortality from pneumonia in children. Because the proportion of cases of ARI receiving medical attention varies so widely among sub-Saharan African countries (6 to 65 percent of such episodes in the four countries mentioned above), it is impossible to estimate the mortality effect of such care-seeking. It is also likely that the diagnosis and treatment of pneumonia by health providers is suboptimal because of limitations in the availability of trained personnel and antibiotics. Given the successful demonstration of the ARI case-management strategy, which emphasizes early detection of pneumonia cases and appropriate antibiotic treatment, it is likely that such programs could have a much greater effect on child mortality than they do now. However, most sub-Saharan African countries have not yet developed ARI control programs, and those countries with programs have just begun their implementation.

SUMMARY

Acute respiratory infections, especially pneumonia, are among the leading causes of death of children in sub-Saharan Africa. The incidence rate in Africa is about 21 per 100 child-years, with the highest incidence observed among the youngest children in households. Most cases of ARI are attributable to two bacteria and the recommended case management is based on antibiotic therapy. Many countries have begun national strategies for combating ARI in recent years. However, there have been few large-scale studies of this approach. A meta-analysis of case-management intervention trials estimated a reduction of infant mortality rate of 15.9 per 1,000 and an under-5 mortality rate reduction of 36 per 1,000. The proportion of children displaying symptoms of ARI who receive medical attention varies by country (from 6 to 65 percent in four DHS in sub-Saharan Africa), and we have little information on current levels of treatment with antibiotics even among those treated at a health clinic. However, given what is known about current levels of antibiotic treatment for ARI, health programs in sub-Saharan Africa probably are not having much effect on overall mortality rates.

5

Nutrition and Nutrition Programs

INTRODUCTION

The synergistic interactions between nutritional status and infectious diseases are an important part of the ecology of disease in Africa. These interactions complicate the evaluation of the effects of health programs because individual disease episodes cannot be treated as independent events. Preventing or treating a disease episode might reduce its nutritional effect, which in turn could reduce the severity of the next disease episode. Because the later episode might involve a different disease than the earlier one, a program to prevent or treat one disease could have implications for mortality due to other diseases. Therefore, health programs might be able to reduce mortality by employing two complementary approaches: preventing or treating infections, and preventing or treating malnutrition.

The term malnutrition often implies one particular nutritional deficiency: protein-energy malnutrition, PEM, which results from inadequate consumption of calories or protein. However, deficiencies of numerous vitamins and other nutrients can be equally serious. It is often difficult to determine which is the major cause of malnutrition: inadequate consumption of specific nutrients (e.g., protein, vitamin A, or iron) or consumption of inadequate quantities of food (usually measured in calories).

This section examines programs designed to reduce the prevalence of protein-energy malnutrition, low birthweight, and vitamin A deficiency. Although other nutritional deficiencies might be equally important, these are the problems most frequently addressed by current program options. We have limited this review to studies that examine whether these interventions reduce mortality in children.

PROTEIN-ENERGY MALNUTRITION (PEM)

PEM can result from inadequate or inappropriate intake of energy, protein, or one or more essential amino acids. It also may be due to temporarily decreased dietary intake resulting from anorexia or malabsorption of nutrients. Many infectious diseases, especially diarrhea, threaten a child's nutritional status by decreasing appetite or reducing the ability to absorb nutrients. In addition, the immunological responses to infection increase nutritional requirements.

Severe PEM can impair a child's response to infectious assaults. For an infection to occur, a pathogen has to overcome the host's immune system. Malnutrition can weaken these defense mechanisms. For example, children with severe clinical malnutrition (kwashiorkor, characterized by lethargy, edema, and dermatitis; and marasmus, characterized by severe wasting associated with depletion of fat and muscle reserves) are more susceptible to gastrointestinal infections because of a reduction in gastric acid (Gracey et al., 1977). PEM also can slow the speed with which an immunological response occurs and can reduce the rate of epithelial replication and tissue repair. Therefore, malnourished children may have longer, more severe cases of what might otherwise be simple childhood infections. In addition, deficiencies in tissue repair may be especially problematic with mucosal surfaces, as in the nasal tract and the intestine. This phenomenon can increase the child's risk of new infections.

Mild to moderate PEM is marked by growth retardation and reduced motor activity. However, most research on PEM now relies on standardized ratios among weight, height, and age. The most commonly used anthropometric indices are height-for-age (Ht/Age), weight-for-height (Wt/Ht), and weight-for-age (Wt/Age). In addition, indices such as upper arm circumference-for-age and -for-height are used to assess nutritional status. There are several ways of comparing these ratios to international standards. The Gomez classification (Gomez et al., 1956) compares a child's weight to a standard schedule of expected weight for a given age. The Waterlow (1972) classification differentiates between stunting (low Ht/Age) and wasting (low Wt/Ht). Stunting results from long-term nutritional insult. Wasting, on the other hand, is a measure of acute undernutrition. Low Wt/Age can result from either stunting or wasting. A child who is two standard deviations (s.d.) below the reference population median for any of the three indexes is classified as undernourished (Hamill et al., 1977; Administrative Committee on Coordination—Subcommittee on Nutrition, United Nations, 1987).

Most early anthropometric studies used the Harvard reference population for comparison (as given in Jelliffe, 1966). More recent studies use the National Center for Health Statistics (NCHS) reference population for comparison (Hamill et al., 1977).

National surveys of nutritional status in sub-Saharan Africa show wide variation in the prevalence of malnutrition, based on the three commonly used indices. Figure 5-1 presents estimates of the proportions with low Wt/Age from the Demographic and Health Surveys (DHS) in eight African countries. Malnutrition tends to be lower during the first year of life, when breastfeeding is more common, than in later years. In fact, in most studies in Africa, children less than 3 months of age are on average heavier than the standard. This finding probably results from excessive mortality rates among low-birthweight infants. From 6 to 23 months of age, malnutrition becomes more common as children experience repeated bouts of diarrhea and other childhood diseases.

Figures 5-2 and 5-3 present age patterns of stunting and wasting. The prevalence of wasting (acute malnutrition) peaks during the second year of

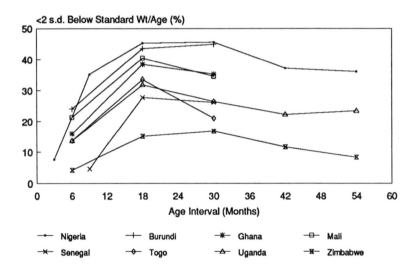

FIGURE 5-1 Prevalence of children malnourished (low weight-for-age) by age of child, sub-Saharan African countries. NOTE: Intervals during first year of life vary by country: Burundi, Ghana, Mali, and Zimbabwe: 3-11 months; Togo and Uganda: 0-11 months; Senegal: 6-11 months; Nigeria: 0-5 and 6-11 months. Intervals after first year of life are: 12-23 months (shown as 18 months), 24-35 months (shown as 30 months), 36-47 months (shown as 42 months), and 48-60 months (shown as 54 months). SOURCE: Demographic and Health Survey reports (see Appendix B).

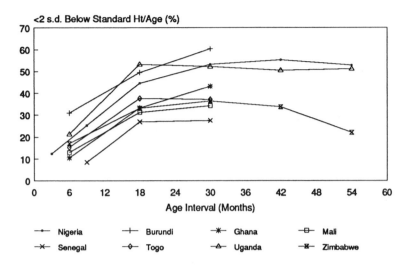

FIGURE 5-2 Prevalence of stunting (low height-for-age) by age of child, sub-Saharan African countries. NOTE: Intervals during first year of life vary by country: Burundi, Ghana, Mali, and Zimbabwe: 3-11 months; Togo and Uganda: 0-11 months; Senegal: 6-11 months;   Nigeria: 0-5 and 6-11 months. Intervals after first year of life are: 12-23 months (shown as 18 months), 24-35 months (shown as 30 months), 36-47 months (shown as 42 months), and 48-60 months (shown as 54 months). SOURCE: Demographic and Health Survey reports (see Appendix B).

life, with national levels for this age group ranging from about 2 to 16 percent. The accumulation of these deficits in growth leads to high levels of stunting among children over age 18 months. The proportions stunted at ages 24-35 months (shown as 30 months on the figure) varies from 28 percent in Senegal to 60 percent in Burundi.

National estimates of the prevalence of malnutrition hide large variations in the prevalence among regions or among social, cultural, and economic groups. Figure 5-4 shows regional estimates of the prevalence of stunting at ages 6-35 months from the DHS in West Africa. Estimates for Togo range from 27 percent stunted in the southern Maritime Region to 48 percent in the northern Savanes Region. Ghana and Nigeria show a similar pattern of higher levels of stunting in the north. In western Mali, the proportion stunted is very similar to neighboring Senegal. The eastern and northern parts of Mali have higher levels of stunting. These regional patterns reflect ecological zones that transcend national boundaries.

The prevalence of malnutrition can vary substantially over quite short distances and among social and ethnic groups. For example, a survey in

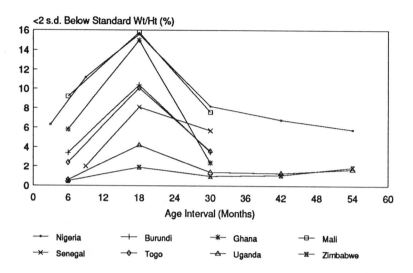

FIGURE 5-3 Prevalence of wasting (low weight-for-height) by age of child, sub-Saharan African countries. NOTE: Intervals during first year of life vary by country: Burundi, Ghana, Mali, and Zimbabwe: 3-11 months; Togo and Uganda: 0-11 months; Senegal: 6-11 months; Nigeria: 0-5 and 6-11 months. Intervals after first year of life are: 12-23 months (shown as 18 months), 24-35 months (shown as 30 months), 36-47 months (shown as 42 months), and 48-60 months (shown as 54 months). SOURCE: Demographic and Health Survey reports (see Appendix B).

northeastern Timbuktu Region of Mali in 1985 after two consecutive crop failures found that 43 percent of nomadic children under age 5 were stunted, compared to only 20 percent of children in sedentary families (Carnell and Guyon, 1990). A study by Mbithi and Wisner (quoted in Kenya Bureau of Statistics, 1979) examined variations in the prevalence of malnutrition among children living on the eastern side of Mt. Kenya. In areas with the best agricultural land at higher altitudes, only 10 percent of children under age 3 years were less than 70 percent of the standard Wt/Age. At lower altitudes, 38 percent of children living in an area with poorer quality agricultural land were below 70 percent of the standard.

Causes of Malnutrition

Malnutrition may arise from a number of conditions, such as lack of food, cessation of breastfeeding, and infection. These factors are often interrelated, making it difficult to determine exactly how a child becomes malnourished.

Food production has not kept pace with population growth in sub-Sa-

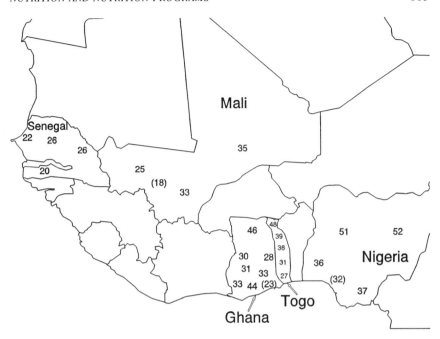

FIGURE 5-4 Proportions of children stunted in regions of Senegal, Mali, Ghana, Togo, and Nigeria.   NOTE: Data for Senegal, Mali (Bamako shown in parentheses), Ghana (Accra shown in parentheses), Togo, and Ondo State, Nigeria (in parentheses) are age standardized, with 42 percent aged 6-17 months and 58 percent aged 18-36 months. The other data for Nigeria are ages 1-59 months. SOURCE: Demographic and Health Survey reports (see Appendix B).

haran Africa. To achieve the needed level of food security, food production in sub-Saharan Africa must grow at about 4 percent per year, but has grown only 2 percent per year since the 1950s (World Bank, 1989).   Drought conditions, lack of infrastructure, and political instability further exacerbate the situation. It is estimated that about 25 percent of the population of sub-Saharan Africa consumes less than 80 percent of the caloric intake recommended by the Food and Agricultural Organization and the World Health Organization (WHO) (World Bank, 1989). Because studies of caloric intake tend to be of limited value due to the difficulty in determining the quantity and nutritional content of foods that are eaten, they are not reviewed here.

Among infants, poor breastfeeding patterns may lead to malnutrition. Breastfeeding is very prevalent for long periods in sub-Saharan Africa. Table 5-1 presents data from the DHS in sub-Saharan Africa on mean duration of breastfeeding and the proportion still breastfeeding during the first two

TABLE 5-1 Breastfeeding Patterns in Sub-Saharan Africa

Country	Mean Duration (months)	Breastfed Child During First Two Months of Life (%)	Breastfed Child Beyond First Year (%)
Botswana	18.8	90.8	73.0
Burundi	23.8	97.0	91.3
Ghana	20.4	92.7	87.2
Kenya	19.4	96.0	81.7
Liberia	17.0	93.4	60.9
Malawi	21.6	90.4	81.5
Nigeria	20.1	96.9	88.4
Senegal	18.8	89.0	86.0
Togo	22.6	95.4	84.2
Uganda	18.6	90.9	84.7
Zimbabwe	19.3	95 .0	87.6

SOURCE: Demographic and Health Survey reports (see Appendix B).

months of life and beyond the first year of life. Mean duration is among the longest in the world, with a range of 17.0 to 23.8 months. Although duration is long, it does not mean that all children are breastfed. The table shows that in all the countries of sub-Saharan Africa included in the DHS (with the exception of Senegal), more than 90 percent of the children are breastfed during the first two months of life. After the first birthday, the proportion still breastfeeding ranged from 61 to 91 percent. Despite the common practice of breastfeeding, it is not uncommon for mothers to stop when their children become ill. Thus, the cessation of breastfeeding may enhance the possibility that an already-sick child will become malnourished, thereby increasing the probability of death.

Infection is one of the common underlying causes of malnutrition. Measles, for example, puts many children below the local standard for Wt/Age and Wt/Ht in the Kasongo Project (1986). Rowland et al. (1977) found that gastroenteritis contributed significantly to growth faltering among Gambian children ages 6 to 35 months, reducing height gain at a rate of 4.2 millimeters per month and weight gain by 746 grams per month, compared to the growth that occurred among unaffected children. Malaria, although much less prevalent than gastroenteritis in the study, reduced weight gain by 1,072 grams per month.

Another study conducted in The Gambia by Rowland et al. (1988) examined Wt/Age among children to assess the relationship between growth and morbidity during the first two years of life. During their first six months, the children exceeded the NCHS reference (see Hamill et al., 1977).

However, during the second six months of life, they had an average deficit of 1.2 kilograms. Rowland et al. attributed the weight faltering principally to diarrhea and acute lower respiratory infections (ALRIs). Diarrhea was responsible for one-half of the deficit (14.4 grams per day among weaning infants) and ALRI for one-fourth (14.7 grams per day of infection).

In a study of growth faltering among Sudanese children, diarrhea was an initiating factor in about 50 percent of cases of faltering (Zumrawi et al., 1987). Among children ages 3 to 6 months, one day of diarrhea reduced the average weight gain of 18 grams to an average loss of 13 grams, a net loss of 31 grams compared to the normal weight change. Colds and cough were associated with a loss of 16 grams per day compared to the normal weight change.

These studies suggest that many common childhood infectious diseases can contribute to growth faltering and malnutrition.

Studies of Malnutrition and Mortality in Other Regions

Several studies have demonstrated that malnourished children are at increased risk of death. For example, Schroeder and Brown (personal communication, 1992) reviewed anthropometric studies in India, Bangladesh, and Papua New Guinea. They examined the relative risk of mortality of children identified as malnourished during the 6- to 24-month period after diagnosis. They concluded that mildly or moderately malnourished children aged 6 to 60 months had a risk of death 2.1 times that of well-nourished children. Severely malnourished children had a risk of dying 6.5 times that of well-nourished children.

The amount of excess risk associated with a given level of malnutrition varies across ecological and social environments. After reviewing a number of studies, Pelletier (1991) concluded that the response of mortality to malnutrition is a function of the baseline level of mortality, with malnutrition having a exacerbating effect on child mortality for any level and type of morbidity that exists in a population.

Studies of the Relationship Among PEM, Morbidity, and Mortality in Africa

The relationship between nutritional status and mortality might be different in Africa than in Asia and Latin America. First, the attributable risk associated with malnutrition (i.e., the extent to which mortality would decline if all children had the mortality rates of well-nourished children) depends on both the percentage malnourished and the degree of malnutrition. If the distribution of children by nutritional status is different in Africa than elsewhere, the attributable risk associated with malnutrition could be different as well. This variation could be true even if the risks associated with various levels of malnutrition are the same in Africa as elsewhere.

Second, in some surveys, nutritional status may serve as a marker for social class. If studies do not control adequately for other risk factors associated with social class, such as education or residence, the estimates of the importance of malnutrition might be exaggerated. It is possible that the link between nutritional status and social class is less important in Africa than in Asia (Bairagi et al., 1985). Third, malaria is a more significant factor in morbidity and mortality in Africa than in most other regions. The interactions between malarial infection and malnutrition are complex and have not been investigated adequately.

PEM and Morbidity

A few studies have examined the link between malnutrition and morbidity in sub-Saharan Africa. A study of children in The Gambia (Tomkins et al., 1989) who were between 6 and 35 months of age at the baseline survey found that short and underweight children experienced an excess risk of illness from diarrhea or fever. The differences persisted after controlling for social, economic, and environmental conditions that might confound the association between the anthropometric index and the excess risk of morbidity.

In the Malumfashi study in Nigeria, however, Tomkins and colleagues (Tomkins, 1981; Tomkins et al., 1991) found that malnutrition had relatively little impact on the incidence of diarrhea, but did increase its prevalence and presumably the average duration of illness.

In the Sudan, El Samani et al. (1988) studied the association between malnutrition and diarrheal disease by weighing and measuring a group of children under age 5 every two months. They reported that children who had experienced an episode of diarrhea in the preceding two months and who were less than 90 percent of the Wt/Age based on the NCHS standard were more likely to have a subsequent diarrheal attack. Among those children who had not had an attack of diarrhea in the preceding two months, the incidence of diarrhea in the subsequent interval was higher among children with Ht/Age less than 95 percent of the standard. After controlling for a number of potentially confounding factors, El Samani et al. found that children with Wt/Age less than 75 percent of the standard were twice as likely to have diarrhea in the subsequent interval, regardless of whether they had had diarrhea in the preceding interval.

Biritwum et al. (1986) found that children in Ghana with Wt/Age less than 80 percent of the WHO standard had a mean of 2.6 episodes of diarrhea per year compared to only 1.7 for other children. This difference was significant at the 95 percent level.

Lang et al. (1986) examined the association between ALRI and nutritional status in Burkina Faso. They found that children with a small arm circumference had a higher incidence and a longer duration of ALRI.

The relationship between nutritional status and morbidity is complex and not well documented in Africa. However, it does appear that malnutrition probably increases the proportion of time a child suffers from diarrhea and may also complicate acute respiratory infections (ARIs).

PEM and Mortality

Lindskog et al. (1988) examined survival rates during the year following an anthropometric survey of children under age 5 in a rural area of Malawi. After adjusting for age, there was a consistent, significant relationship between mortality and nutritional status as measured by height-for-age, weight-for-height, or weight-for-age. For example, as shown in Table 5-2, children who were between 1 and 2 standard deviations below the standard Ht/Age had a relative risk of death 1.46 times that of children with a higher Ht/Age. Those who were more than four standard deviations below the standard had a relative risk of 3.3.

The Kasongo Project (1983) in Zaire observed that the risk of mortality was 1.8 times greater among children with Wt/Age indices less than 80 percent of the Harvard standard median (see Jelliffe, 1966) than among other children. Those less than 60 percent of the median were 3.3 times more likely to die than better-nourished children. (They did not present confidence intervals or significance tests for these differences.) These risk ratios were lower than the values the authors reported based on the data for India provided by Kielmann and McCord (1978).

TABLE 5-2 Effect on Relative Risk Estimates of Controlling for Age and Period on the Relationship Between Height-for-Age and Child Mortality, Malawi, 1983-1985

Ht/Age Score (standard deviations from median)	Raw Relative Risks	Adjusted Relative Risks
Greater than -1 s.d.	1.00	1.00
-2 to -1 s.d.	0.88	1.46
-3 to -2 s.d.	0.76	1.71
-4 to -3 s.d.	1.15	2.79
Less than -4 s.d.	1.07	3.30

NOTE: Adjustments are made by introducing age (0-5, 6-11, 12-17, 18-23, 24-35, 36-39 months) and period into the log-linear regression analysis.

SOURCE: Lindskog et al. (1988).

A study by Smedman et al. (1987) of children aged 6 to 59 months in Guinea-Bissau examined survival during the 8 to 12 months following weighing and measuring. They reported that Ht/Age was correlated with child survival after controlling for the age of the child. However, Wt/Ht was not significantly related to survival. They also noted that their findings showed less effect of nutritional status than studies in Asia.

Briend et al. (1989) examined survival rates for children in rural Senegal during the six months following semiannual weighings. They concluded that survival is related to nutritional status, and the risk is most closely related to muscle mass rather than to the standard nutritional indices.

These studies show that poor nutritional status is associated with higher mortality, although the relationship appears to be weaker than that found in similar studies in Asia. These studies do not prove that the relationship between nutritional status and mortality is causal. Although poor nutritional status may compromise the immune system, it is also possible that poor nutritional status and elevated risk of death are jointly affected by some other unmeasured characteristic of children such as child care practices, access to health care, or differences in socioeconomic class or housing, or by some other aspect of nutritional status such as vitamin A deficiency.

PEM and Measles Mortality

There is solid evidence that children with measles often develop malnutrition (Kasongo Project Team, 1986; Reddy et al., 1986). However, Aaby et al. (1984a-c, 1986) questioned whether malnutrition is associated with higher case-fatality rates for measles.

Many studies (such as Kimati and Lyaruu, 1976) have examined the relationship between nutritional status and case fatality due to measles in hospitals. Generally, however, hospital-based studies cannot provide evidence of the temporal relationship among malnutrition, the onset of measles, and subsequent mortality. For example, many of the severe cases in hospitals are among children who were sick for several days before coming to the hospital. Among these cases, there might be an increased prevalence of low Wt/Age as a result of several days of illness.

There have also been several studies based on long-term monitoring of anthropometry, measles cases, and mortality. For example, a study in Bangladesh (Koster et al., 1981) weighed and measured each child every two months. Children who died of measles had weights and heights comparable to those of controls matched for age, sex, and neighborhood. There was no evidence in the study that preexisting malnutrition increased the risk of death from measles.

Aaby (1992) presented data from a measles epidemic in Bandim, Guinea-

Bissau, in 1979 that showed no difference in case fatality by Wt/Age before the case. The case-fatality rate for children less than 80 percent of the standard Wt/Age was not noticeably different from that of children with Wt/Age 80-99 percent of the standard or more than 100 percent of the standard. There were still no differences after controlling for age and whether the case was the only case in the household (Smedman et al., 1987).

Aaby et al. (1984a) presented data on nutritional status for 44 cases of measles in Quinhamel, Guinea-Bissau, in 1979-1982. The children who died had a mean Wt/Age slightly less than those who survived (86.7 percent of the WHO standard compared to 89.8). However, the difference again was not significant. This approach is not a good way to test the relative risk of death associated with undernutrition. Rather, the approach is more closely related to the issue of the sensitivity of nutritional status for identifying those at risk.

The Machakos study (Muller et al., 1977) compared the upper-arm circumferences (UAC) of those who died of measles with controls matched for age, residence, and measles diagnostic score. The UAC for the deceased was significantly lower than the values for the survivors (81.0 compared to 84.8; probability less than or equal to .05). However, a later analysis demonstrated that this difference disappeared if controls were selected from among the survivors of the same epidemic. Because both nutritional status and case fatality differed between epidemics, the relationship between UAC and case fatality was apparently spurious (Leeuwenburg et al., 1984, as described by Aaby, 1988).

Lamb (1988) did not find a significant effect of nutritional status on either the incidence or the severity of measles infections in an epidemic in The Gambia. However, the sample size was quite small (54 cases), and it is not clear how many children were weighed in the weeks preceding their case of measles.

The Kasongo Project Team (1983) showed that the distribution of measles cases by nutritional status was not very different from that of all deaths. Therefore, they did not present a separate analysis of measles deaths.

The relationship between nutritional status and the case-fatality rate for measles remains uncertain in Africa. All of the studies are hindered by several differences between Africa and Asia. First, the levels of malnutrition are relatively low in many parts of Africa compared to Asia. Any effect of nutritional status is apt to be most pronounced at the most severe levels of malnutrition. Therefore, the relationship between nutritional status and case fatality may be smaller in African than in Asia. Second, any analysis must control for the difference in case fatality between primary and secondary cases of measles because compound households, where a larger proportion of cases are likely to be secondary, are very common in much of Africa.

Finally, it is not clear what constitutes the most important aspect of nutritional status in determining mortality risks. If vitamin A deficiency is the most important mechanism, the standard anthropometric indices may show a strong relationship to survival only if the occurrence of PEM is a good marker for vitamin A deficiency. It is possible that the relationship between PEM and vitamin A status is different in Africa than in other regions.

All of these factors suggest that it would require a large sample size to determine the effect of nutritional status on measles case fatality in Africa. For example, by using a case-fatality rate of 18 percent among well-nourished cases (slightly less than the 20 percent among all cases in Bandim) and a relative risk of 2 for the worst 10 percent of the population, a sample size of 540 would be required to have a power of 80 percent. This number is twice the sample size available for the largest analysis in Bandim. Controlling for differences between single cases in a household and secondary cases, as well as for age, would increase the required sample size.

Studies of the Effect of Nutrition Programs on Mortality in Africa

The existence of excess mortality among malnourished children does not prove that programs addressing nutritional status will reduce child mortality. If the relationship between malnutrition and mortality is not causal (direct or indirect), then merely changing nutritional status may not change mortality.

Interventions designed to improve nutritional status of mothers and children are typically based on one or more of the following: supplementary feeding, growth monitoring, breastfeeding, and weaning education.

Although a number of nutrition interventions have been implemented in sub-Saharan Africa, few have been evaluated scientifically. One study, the Iringa Nutrition Programme, was conducted in 168 villages of rural Tanzania between 1983 and 1988, and was evaluated between June and October 1988 (Chorlton, 1989). The Iringa Nutrition Programme was a community-development program that included subprojects related to maternal and child health, water and environmental sanitation, household food security, and income-generating activities. Over the course of the study, the percentage of children aged 1 to 60 months that were underweight (i.e., less than 80 percent of the Harvard standard for Wt/Age) decreased from about 48 to 37 percent. The percentage of children seriously underweight (less than 60 percent of the standard Wt/Age) declined from about 5 to less than 2 percent. A comparison of the percentage of children seriously undernourished who lived in villages not included in the program indicated a prevalence of 5.6 percent during August-October 1987, which was close to the 6.3 percent prevalence in the study area when the study began.

The mortality data from the Iringa Nutrition Programme include the number and proportion of deaths due to specific causes. Over the course of the study, deaths from respiratory infections and diarrhea were reported to have decreased, measles deaths were fairly constant, and deaths from fever (presumably malaria) increased. However, it is not possible to estimate death rates based on the data provided, because the authors did not supply adequate information on exposure to death. Were it possible to estimate age-specific rates from the data, the study would be more helpful in determining the effect of nutritional status on mortality.

The team that evaluated the Iringa Nutrition Programme concluded that these data provide a strong indication of the program's effect. However, the lack of a control area made it difficult to reach such a conclusion. Moreover, the evaluation did not classify children as stunted or wasted, nor did it provide data by age.

Perhaps hundreds of small- and large-scale nutrition programs have been undertaken in different parts of Africa. In a qualitative review of the factors contributing to successful nutrition programs in the region, Kennedy (1991) discussed seven key elements: community participation, program flexibility, institutional structure, recovery of recurrent costs, multifaceted program activities, well-trained and qualified staff, and the presence of infrastructure. However, because most nutrition programs do not gather mortality data, it is not possible to conclude much about the effect of these programs on survival.

Supplementary Feeding Programs

Beaton and Ghassemi (1982) reviewed the effect of supplementary feeding programs on nutritional status and reported that such programs should improve nutritional status of children, but often do not because of low coverage, low levels of supplementation, food sharing, and food substitution.

Few programs collect data on the morbidity (other than relief of malnutrition itself) and mortality consequences of food supplementation programs. Studies in Guatemala, India, and Peru found a significant reduction in infant and/or child mortality due to supplementary feeding alone (Ascoli et al., 1967; Scrimshaw et al., 1968; Baertl et al., 1970; Kielmann and McCord, 1978). However, no evidence of such effects of programs implemented in Africa was uncovered.

Growth Monitoring

Monitoring the growth of infants and children may increase the effect of programs that provide nutrition rehabilitation or other services that can be targeted to malnourished children. In Jamaica, a reduction in mortality was observed following increased access to primary health care in association with growth monitoring and targeted provision of food (Alderman et al., 1978). However, this program was tested in an area with mortality rates comparable to the lowest rates in Africa—mortality at ages 1-48 months of 14.5 deaths per 1,000 before the start of the program.

In Malawi (Cole-King, 1975), there was a decline in the proportion malnourished following the expansion of the national system of under-5 clinics. The percentage of undernourished children (based on the Wt/Age index) dropped from 37 in the first year to 29 percent in the second and third years. However, the clinics offered a wide range of services in addition to growth monitoring, so it is not possible to determine what part of the change in nutritional status might have been caused by nutrition activities.

The potential effect of growth monitoring programs is limited by the sensitivity and specificity of nutritional status as a screening tool for identifying those with the highest risk of death. For example, the Kasongo Project Team (1983) emphasized that the sensitivities of the various anthropometric measures are very low. Their data suggest that if a program in Kasongo targeted children below the tenth percentile in Wt/Age using a local standard and reduced their mortality rate to the average for other children, mortality would drop by only about 10 percent.

These calculations suggest that even if a program succeeded in eliminating all the excess mortality associated with malnutrition, the effect on mortality would be so small that it would be hard to measure. Although some other areas of Africa have a higher prevalence of low Wt/Age than Kasongo, it would still be difficult to measure the effects of the most successful programs.

Studies that have examined the effect of growth monitoring have found little benefit. At a recent UNICEF meeting, it was suggested that growth monitoring not be adopted as a global strategy, but that growth promotion should be. Weighing or measuring all children is a difficult undertaking and the information is often used inappropriately by individuals, households, or communities. Thus, UNICEF has developed a three-step program for growth promotion strategies, which includes activities such as nutrition education, surveillance, and paying special attention to children identified as high risk in community-based nutrition surveillance (United Nations Children's Fund, 1992).

Programs Designed to Change Breastfeeding and Weaning

Weaning education can modify behavior, but it must address the cultural norms and social and economic conditions of the groups to which it is directed. Several strategies have been shown to result in improved nutritional status in sub-Saharan Africa. These include rehabilitation centers for malnourished children in Zaire (Brown and Brown, 1979); home-based training of mothers in various aspects of food production and preparation, food hygiene, and basic health care in Uganda (Hoorveg and McDowell, 1979); and community-based activities such as demonstrations and group lessons on low-cost, homemade, weaning foods carried out by village-based volunteer monitors in Burkina Faso (Zeitlin, 1981). These studies showed improvements in nutritional status of children, but did not assess the effects on mortality. Weaning education may also contribute to a reduction in mortality from other causes in which malnutrition is a complicating factor.

The promotion of breastfeeding is another type of nutrition intervention that is related to improved probability of child survival. Breastfeeding ensures that a child receives adequate nutrition in early infancy. Moreover, it protects the child from diarrhea, ARI, and other diseases (Feachem and Koblinsky, 1984; Huffman et al., 1991).

Strategies for increasing the initiation and duration of exclusive breastfeeding include training and education of health professionals (Potter et al., 1987), changes in hospital practices that facilitate immediate initiation (Klaus and Kennel, 1976), keeping mother and child in the same room (Mata, 1983), and restriction of infant formula samples (Bergevin et al., 1983). Although a number of studies have examined the effect of breastfeeding on nutritional status and disease prevention, they generally do not measure its effect on mortality.

LOW BIRTHWEIGHT

Low birthweight (LBW), typically defined as weighing less than 2,500 grams at birth, has been reported to be the strongest predictor of infant mortality, especially in the neonatal period (Susser et al., 1972). LBW appears to affect mortality through direct and indirect mechanisms. Children with the condition are more likely to have impaired cellular immunity, which may increase their risk of early cases of diarrhea, respiratory infection, and other infections.

Studies of the Relationship Between Low Birthweight and Mortality

The increased risk of mortality among LBW infants has been demonstrated in a number of studies in other regions (Shapiro, 1968; Puffer and Serrano, 1973; De Vaquera et al., 1983; Victora et al., 1988). There are few similar studies in Africa.

Mbacké and van de Walle (1992) examined the role of birthweight on survival using a cohort study of all births in maternity hospitals in the town of Bobo-Dioulasso, Burkina Faso, between April 1981 and March 1984. They reported neonatal, postneonatal, and second-year death rates by birthweight for 6,091 births who either survived to age 2 years or died before that age. More than 13 percent of these children had birthweights less than 2,500 grams. The infant mortality rate for these low-birthweight infants was 3.88 times (95 percent confidence interval (C.I.) 3.32-4.54) the rate among births with weights greater than 2,500 grams (250 and 64.4 per 1,000 live births).[1] Extending the analysis through the second year of life reduces the relative risk somewhat. The risk of dying before age 2 years was 2.84 times (95 percent C.I. 2.48-3.24) as high for low-birthweight children as for other children. (The probability of dying by age 2, $_2q_0$, were 285 and 101 per 1,000 live births.)

Mbacké and van de Walle also tested whether the difference in postneonatal and second-year mortality rates remained after controlling for socioeconomic factors (father's income, mother's education, type of home, etc.) and other risk factors (sex, twins, month of birth, birth order, housing density, number and timing of prenatal visits, and use of measures against malaria). They found that those children with weights greater than 3,000 grams still had a postneonatal mortality rate significantly lower than low-birthweight children (odds ratio of 0.53; probability less that or equal to .001), and those weighing 2,500-2,599 grams still had a lower postneonatal mortality rate than low-birthweight children (odds ratio of 0.84; not significant). After controlling for other factors, there was no significant difference by birthweight in the second-year mortality rate.

Low birthweight is a relatively common condition. It is estimated that approximately 17 percent of all births in developing countries are LBW (World Health Organization, 1980). The condition varies a lot by region, with higher prevalence observed in Asia and lower prevalence in Latin America and Africa (World Health Organization, 1980a). The underlying cause of LBW is also different when less and more developed countries are compared. Intrauterine growth retardation is estimated to account for more than half of LBW infants in developing countries, whereas preterm delivery is the major cause of LBW in developed countries (Kramer, 1987).

The prevalence of LBW in many sub-Saharan African countries is unknown because of unattended births and poor registration systems. In the Machakos study in Kenya, 7.0 percent of the births were LBW (Muller and van Ginneken, 1991). In a study of the effect of malaria prophylaxis on birthweight in Burkina Faso, the incidence of LBW was 16.4 percent for both the test and the control groups (Cot et al., 1992). There are several studies of birthweight among births in African hospitals. However, hospital births may not provide an unbiased sample of all births. Although the

---

[1]These estimates are based on the data presented by Mbacké and van de Walle (1992:132).

prevalence of LBW in sub-Saharan Africa exceeds that of developed countries, it may be lower than that observed in Asia (Kramer, 1987).

Risk Factors for Low Birthweight

A number of factors, such as inadequate prenatal care, inadequate maternal weight gain, physically demanding work, short birth intervals, and tobacco or alcohol consumption have been associate with LBW. These conditions can be modified through interventions prior to or during pregnancy. These types of factors tend to be correlated with LBW, but may not cause it. LBW and factors such as inadequate prenatal care and short birth intervals may be jointly influenced by unobserved characteristics such as access to health care and socioeconomic status.[2] Other factors, such as multiple births, maternal height, and birth order also affect birthweight, but are not as easily addressed through interventions.

Physically Demanding Work

Two studies in Africa suggest that a seasonal increase in the energy expenditure of pregnant women may affect birthweight more than a seasonal decrease in caloric intake. The Keneba study in The Gambia noted a decrease in birthweight preceding the decrease in seasonal intake and paralleling the increase in physical work (Roberts et al., 1982). Similarly, a study in Tanzania did not see any seasonal decrease in birthweight when rains delayed the beginning of field work (Bantje, 1983).

Short Birth Intervals

One of the motives for family planning programs has been the promotion of longer birth intervals to reduce the prevalence of LBW. The Demographic and Health Surveys conducted in sub-Saharan Africa reinforce the strength of the association between short birth intervals and infant mortality. Figure 5-5 illustrates that as birth intervals become longer, perhaps through the use of contraceptives, the infant mortality rate decreases, although the analysis does not control for any potential confounding factors.

This negative association between short birth intervals and survival has been widely studied (e.g., Hobcraft et al., 1985), but the biological mechanism is not well understood. The relationship between socioeconomic status and birth intervals might explain part of the apparent effect of intervals

---

[2]Biased estimates may result in estimating the effects of prenatal care or birth intervals on birthweight if improper procedures are used. See Rosenzweig and Schultz (1983) and Schultz (1984) for further discussion of this bias and procedures for minimizing it.

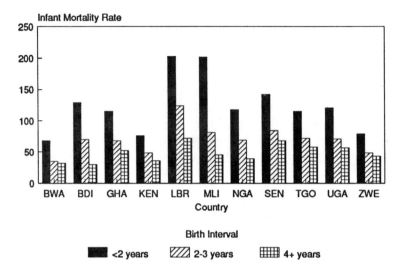

FIGURE 5-5 Infant mortality rate by length of preceding birth interval. NOTE: BWA—Botswana, BDI—Burundi, GHA—Ghana, KEN-Kenya, LBR—Liberia, MLI-Mali, NGA—Nigeria, SEN—Senegal, TGO-Togo, UGA—Uganda, ZWE—Zimbabwe. SOURCE: Demographic and Health Survey reports (see Appendix B).

on mortality. We do not have any evidence of how much infant mortality might be reduced by changes in breastfeeding and contraceptive use that increase birth intervals.

Prenatal Care

Studies in Nigeria (Oruamabo and John, 1989; Wright, 1990) report that prenatal care is associated with a lower risk of LBW because some of the biological factors that contribute to the condition can be controlled or monitored through regular medical attention.

Onyemunwa (1988) reported that in a study of Nigerian women, the majority (92 percent) of the women received at least one prenatal visit. However, the significant association with infant mortality was the timing of initiating prenatal care. Women who began receiving care during the sixth month of pregnancy or later were 48 percent more likely to experience the death of the child than those women who began prenatal care during the first through fifth months. However, it may be that some unmeasured variable was responsible for both the use of prenatal care and child death.

Results from the DHS in sub-Saharan Africa indicate that the use of prenatal care varies across countries. Figure 5-6 shows that in most coun-

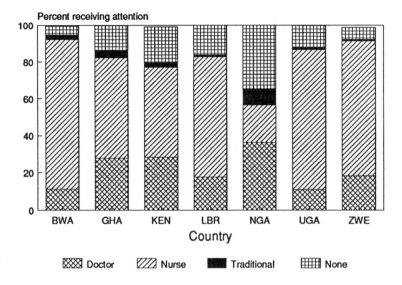

FIGURE 5-6 Prenatal care received in pregnencies over previous five years, select-
ed countries of sub-Saharan Africa. NOTE: BWA—Botswana, GHA—Ghana, KEN-
Kenya, LBR—Liberia, NGA—Nigeria, UGA—Uganda, ZWE—Zimbabwe. SOURCE:
Demographic and Health Survey reports (see Appendix B).

tries, the majority of women report some prenatal care from either a doctor
or a nurse. In Nigeria and Mali, however, 35 and 62 percent, respectively,
did not receive any prenatal care.[3]   We do not know whether the number or
timing of the visits or the type of advice given or heeded was sufficient to
have any impact on the outcome of pregnancies or child survival.

Malaria

As discussed earlier, malarial infections in pregnant women are associated with increased risk of low birthweight (McGregor, 1984; Greenwood et
al., 1989; Cot et al., 1992).   This problem is most common among first
births (McGregor, 1984; Greenwood et al., 1989).   It is not clear what
proportion of LBW in Africa is attributable to malaria.   However, it may be
the cause that can be addressed most successfully by health programs.   Programs to address malaria during pregnancy are reviewed in Chapter 4.

---

[3]In most countries, a few percentage of women reported receiving prenatal care from a
traditional birth attendant or someone else.   In Liberia, 17.1 percent reported another source.

Effects of Programs on the Incidence of Low Birthweight

There are a number of studies that examine the effect of various interventions on the incidence of low birthweight. Since these studies rarely examine the resulting effect on infant mortality and most are small-scale studies, we have not made a complete survey of all of them. However, it is useful to mention a few to indicate the types of programs that have been tested and the conclusions reached.

Small-scale studies of pregnant women have reported significant improvements in birthweights from nutrition supplementation. A study in Guatemala (Lechtig et al., 1975a,b) examined the effect of two supplements (one with high protein and caloric value, the other with a lower caloric value and no protein). The infants of the better-supplemented group had a mean birthweight that was 111 grams higher than the poorly supplemented group. The prevalence of LBW was 17 percent in the poorly supplemented group and 8 percent in the better-supplemented group. The study also demonstrated that caloric intake rather than protein appears to be the principal factor limiting fetal development. It also suggested that the total additional calories consumed during pregnancy appear to have been more important than the calories consumed during the trimester when supplementation was begun.

In the village of Keneba in The Gambia, a food supplementation program for pregnant women produced a significant increase in birthweight (Prentice, 1983; Prentice et al., 1987). Women were given biscuits and fortified tea six days a week, providing 950 calories per day during the dry season and 1,110 calories per day during the wet season when food was less plentiful. Moreover, the supplement tasted good and was offered early in the morning when most of the women would not normally have eaten at home. Among the inadequately nourished mothers, the supplementation increased the mean birthweight by 225 grams and decreased the prevalence of LBW from 28 to 5 percent—a reduction of 82 percent. Among all women, the increase in birthweight was 120 grams, and a 68 percent reduction in the percentage of LBW infants was observed.

VITAMIN A DEFICIENCY

Vitamin A deficiency is widespread in developing regions of the world, especially Africa and Asia. The condition results in a number of health disorders and is often manifested in problems with the eye and vision. Vitamin A has important functions in the human body. One of its physiological functions is in the formation and maintenance of epithelial tissue, which contributes to the body's immune system. Vitamin A is essential to growth of the skin as well as the mucous membranes lining the ocular and oral cavities, and the respiratory, genitourinary, and gastrointestinal tracts. When vitamin A is deficient, the epithelial cells become dry and flat, hardening so that absorption of nutrients is reduced. Moreover, vitamin A deficiency may increase the risk of bacterial colonization or delay recovery.

It is estimated that each year, approximately 10 million cases of childhood xerophthalmia (dryness of the conjunctiva and cornea) occur worldwide, with more than 500,000 resulting in blindness (Feachem, 1987). Vitamin A deficiency is often associated with specific regions of the world, such as Africa and Asia, where diets often lack carotene-containing foods.

Studies of Vitamin A Deficiency, Morbidity, and Mortality

The lack of data makes it difficult to assess the prevalence of vitamin A deficiency for sub-Saharan Africa or for individual countries. However, a few studies in sub-Saharan Africa provide some estimates. In the Lower Shire River Valley of Malawi, for example, 5.4 percent of children less than 6 years of age experienced night blindness and 3.9 percent of children suffered active corneal disease (Tielsch et al., 1986). In southern Ethiopia, De Sole et al. (1987) reported an average prevalence of vitamin A deficiency of 5.4 percent in boys aged 6 months to 6 years, and 5.5 percent in girls of the same age.

A few studies in sub-Saharan Africa support the association between vitamin A deficiency and more severe cases of diarrhea, measles, and respiratory infections. In southern Ethiopia, De Sole et al. (1987) reported that the prevalence of severe cases of diarrhea in the previous year was twice as high among children with vitamin A deficiency as among children without the deficit.

A number of studies have indicated that children with severe vitamin A deficiency and xerophthalmia experience elevated rates of mortality. Death rates among children hospitalized with these conditions range on average from 15 to 25 percent (Kuming and Politzer, 1967; Sommer et al., 1975; Brown et al., 1979; Sommer, 1982). Most studies do not attribute the deaths to the deficiency of vitamin A but rather to concurrent illnesses and conditions that are exacerbated by reduced levels of vitamin A, such as PEM, diarrhea, and respiratory infections.

Studies of Vitamin A Supplementation and Mortality Reduction

A number of vitamin A supplementation studies have been conducted, principally in Asia, that demonstrate a positive effect on reducing infant and child mortality. In a meta-analysis of vitamin A supplementation studies conducted in Asia, Tonascia et al. (personal communication, 1992) estimated the weighted reduction in mortality attributable to vitamin A deficiency for children 6 months or older (up to approximately 83 months at follow-up) to be 34 percent. They noted that the magnitude of the effect may depend on the extent and severity of nutritional deficiencies, the cause-of-death structure of infant and child mortality, cultural and environmental factors, and the study design and implementation.

Sommer et al. (1986) conducted a randomized controlled community trial of periodic large-dose vitamin A supplementation in northern Sumatra, Indonesia. During the follow-up period, almost all deaths in program villages were among children who had not received the supplement. Preschool children in the treatment group experienced a 34 percent reduction in the noninfant mortality rates compared to the comparison group. In a reanalysis of the same data, Tarwotjo et al. (1987) reported that among children between ages 3 and 11 months, mortality rates were 0.9 per 1,000 in the treatment group, compared to 12.0 in the nontreatment group and 6.0 in the control areas. They concluded that the 34 percent reduction reported in the previous article may be an underestimate because the early analysis was based on intent to treat (i.e., results for all children allocated to one regimen are compared with those allocated to the other, regardless of whether they received the regimen assigned) at the community level, rather than on those actually receiving the intervention at the individual level. In southern India, Rahmathullah et al. (1990) reported that vitamin A supplements equivalent to the level recommended by international groups, when given on a weekly basis, reduced the relative risk of mortality in children under 5 years of age by 54 percent. Mortality rates in the control group were 10.5 per 1,000 compared to 4.8 per 1,000 in the treatment group. West et al. (1991) conducted a trial of the efficacy of vitamin A supplementation in reducing childhood mortality in Nepal. In a randomized, double-blind community trial of almost 29,000 children aged 6-72 months, supplemented children received 60,000 retinol equivalents every four months and the placebo-treated group received 300 retinol equivalents. After 12 months, the relative risk of death among the supplemented group was 70 percent that of the control group, supporting the hypothesis that vitamin A supplementation can contribute to lower overall child mortality. Daulaire et al. (1992) found that the risk of death for Nepali children aged 1 to 59 months in supplemented communities was 26 percent lower than in unsupplemented communities, with the largest reduction of 49 percent among children 6 to 11 months of age.

Although most studies find an association between vitamin A supplementation and a reduction in mortality, a prospective double-blind placebo-controlled study conducted in Hyderabad, India, reported no significant difference when supplementation occurred. The study, conducted by Vijayaraghavan et al. (1990), indicated that mortality rates were similar in the groups receiving the supplement and the placebo.

Herrera et al. (1992) also found no mortality effect in a controlled, masked randomized trial of 29,615 children in northern Sudan where there was a clear association between dietary vitamin A and mortality, based on a nonsignificant difference in the number of deaths between the comparison and treatment groups. In that study, some children were assigned to a group that received 200,000 international units (IU) of vitamin A and 40 IU of vitamin E every six months. The control group received only 40 IU of vitamin E. Over the 18 months of the study, there was no apparent effect of large-dose vitamin A supplementation on mortality. It is not understood why the findings of this study in northern Sudan differ from those conducted in other parts of the world. Perhaps political and social conditions were impediments to the study. On the other hand, the nonsignificant effect of vitamin A supplementation may be based on differing disease epidemiologies due to ecological differences.

For Africa, the most recent evidence on the effect of vitamin A supplementation, morbidity, and mortality comes from an experiment in northern Ghana. There, in an intervention trial among mildly vitamin A-deficient children conducted by Ross et al. (Beaton et al., 1992) a reduction of 20 percent in mortality is reported among the supplemented group compared to the control group (probability less than .003).

SUMMARY

A variety of nutrition-related conditions exacerbate the mortality effect of several diseases. Protein-energy malnutrition, although rare during the first six months of life, is common among children between 6 and 23 months of age, and is associated with increases in diarrheal and other diseases. Wide variations in the prevalence of malnutrition are observed in sub-Saharan Africa, and a number of studies suggest that the effect of nutritional status is less important in Africa than in Asia. Many programs that address malnutrition do not necessarily reduce mortality. Most nutrition interventions do not gather information on mortality. Supplemental feeding programs often do not reach the target populations; growth monitoring may make mothers aware of how their children are developing, but it has little direct effect on reducing mortality.

Mild and severe vitamin A deficiency seems to be associated with excess mortality. Studies conducted principally in Asia report higher overall and cause-specific mortality among children with this deficiency. Again, little evidence exists to make conclusions about the effect of vitamin A supplementation in sub-Saharan Africa.

6

Integrated and General Health Programs

INTRODUCTION

The previous chapters reviewed studies of disease-specific interventions. In practice, few health programs are limited to a single intervention against a single disease. Immunization programs include vaccinations against several diseases (usually tuberculosis, diphtheria, pertussis, tetanus, polio, and measles). Health centers often offer vaccinations, as well as treatment for fever, diarrhea, and tuberculosis, and many provide growth monitoring and health education. Hospitals often include a health center that provides all these services as well as curative services for a wide range of diseases and conditions, including pregnancy.

Integrated services are expected to have an effect on mortality because they generally include some interventions that have demonstrated effects when delivered alone. For example, because most health centers and hospitals provide measles vaccinations, at a minimum these programs have an impact through this one service. However, we would like to know whether the effects of these integrated services are larger than the effects of much simpler (and presumably cheaper) programs based on a few selected interventions.

Integrated health programs, health centers, and hospitals should not be evaluated solely on the basis of their effect on mortality. In the first place, they provide services that reduce morbidity, and they often serve as training centers for doctors and other health personnel. Second, hospitals also have the potential to serve as centers for research into local health problems. Third, the development of efficient health centers and hospitals is a necessary precondition for the continuing improvement of health services in Africa (Mosley, 1988; Newell, 1988). Although many of the individual interventions can be delivered efficiently without extensive investment in health centers and hospitals, that may not be true of the interventions that will be the focus of future efforts to improve health services in Africa (Ewbank and Zimicki, 1988). For example, although vaccinations can be provided through periodic visits of mobile teams, treatment for acute illnesses such as malaria and respiratory infections must be available almost continuously. In addition, as the number of services provided increases, the relative cost-effectiveness of fixed clinics may increase because the fixed costs of the clinic are distributed over a larger number of effective interventions. Therefore, health centers and hospitals should be evaluated in the context of the continuing development of general health services.

Evaluation of the efficacy of integrated health programs is much more problematic than evaluation of single interventions. First, it is difficult to assume that the results of a study of one program apply to other programs because there is substantial variation among integrated programs. For example, some vaccination programs include locally important vaccines such as meningococcal vaccine. Similarly, health centers differ in the number of drugs and amount of equipment available, the staffing patterns, and the skill level of personnel. Even if the same services are offered, there might be substantial variation in the mix of services actually delivered. For example, health centers may encourage mothers to return monthly for the series of diphtheria-pertussis-tetanus (DPT) and polio injections, but may find it difficult to have them return for a measles injection after the child is 9 months old. On the other hand, mobile clinics may achieve higher coverage of measles (a single injection) than DPT, which requires three injections each separated by at least one month.

A second problem in the evaluation of integrated programs is that it is often difficult to identify and maintain control areas. When national programs begin, there is often an attempt to introduce them in all parts of the country as quickly as possible. For example, the evaluation of the Combatting Childhood Communicable Diseases Project in Zaire began with a program area and a control area. However, after the baseline survey, the program managers decided to combine the two areas into one health zone (Chahnazarian et al., 1993).

Even when scientists can define control areas, it is often difficult to limit the use of services to those living in the intervention areas. For example, it is rarely possible to restrict access to a health center to a defined population. Therefore, evaluations of such programs are prone to contamination of the control area.

Finally, the more complex the program, the less likely are all of its aspects to be successfully introduced simultaneously. Therefore, there is no exact date for the start of the program. Training of personnel often continues after the start of services, the range of services may increase slowly, and problems in management and staffing may delay the effective operation of the program. In many cases, the program will be phased in over so many years that it is not feasible to separate its effects from long-term trends.

Given these difficulties, it is not surprising that few studies have produced reliable estimates of the effect of hospitals, health centers, or integrated programs.

CASE STUDIES OF LONG-TERM MORTALITY TRENDS

The best evidence for the effect of health programs on mortality in Africa comes from a few studies of long-term trends in mortality in West Africa. Although these studies do not offer the kind of rigorous proof provided by randomized trials or even natural experiments with control areas, they do suggest that the expansion of health services has had an impact on survival rates.

Mlomp, Senegal

Pison et al. (1993) have examined mortality trends in Mlomp, a rural area in southern Senegal. Maternity histories collected in 1984-1985 were compared with registers from maternity clinics, civil registers, and records from religious missions and health dispensaries. These data provide estimates of infant and child mortality for the period 1930-1984. Although the quality of these estimates cannot match that of a continuous registration system, they provide a reasonable outline of mortality trends. It appears that the proportion of children dying by age 5 was quite stable at about 350-370 per 1,000 from 1930 to 1960. After 1960 mortality began to decline rapidly and fell to only 81 per 1,000 for 1985-1989.

Pison et al. provide a convincing case for the conclusion that this rapid decline in mortality and the very low levels today are due largely to the introduction of health services during the 1960s and 1970s. These services include the opening of a dispensary in 1961 and a maternity clinic in 1968. Vaccination programs started in 1971, but were irregular until the late 1970s. By 1980 most children were correctly vaccinated. Ninety-nine percent of the children born in Mlomp in 1988 and still living in the area had received measles, yellow fever, BCG, DPT, and polio vaccines. A growth monitoring program began in 1969 and supplementary foods were provided to mothers and children. In 1975, an antimalarial program began promoting regular doses of chloroquine during the rainy season. Chloroquine is provided free to pregnant women and young children.

The effect of these programs can be seen in data on cause of death and in epidemiologic data. In 1963 a survey showed a malaria parasite rate of 50 percent in children. In 1989 the prevalence of malaria parasitemia was only 3 percent among children aged 0-6 years at the end of the rainy season. During 1985-1989 the data on cause of death suggest that the probability of dying of malaria between ages 1 month and 5 years was only 2 per 1,000. The last epidemics of measles occurred in 1972 and 1974. During 1985-1989 there were no measles deaths and only one death from whooping cough.

There have been socioeconomic changes in Mlomp, but they were probably not responsible for most of the declines in infant and child mortality rates. Education levels of women have only increased recently, and in 1985-1989 only 26 percent of the births were to mothers who had completed at least one year of schooling. Transportation improved, but not until after the mortality decline was well established. Finally, there was no substantial improvement in the economic situation in the area.

The Mlomp example suggests that the provision of basic health services can bring about substantial declines in infant and child mortality.

Keneba, The Gambia, 1950-1984

Four villages (Keneba, Manduar, Jali, Kanton-Kunda) located in the West-Kiang district in The Gambia, totaling about 2,000 persons, have been followed by a team of British researchers since 1949 (Billewicz and McGregor, 1982; Lamb et al., 1984). During the first 25 years, there was no evidence of mortality decline in Keneba. If anything there was a small rise in mortality from 1950 until 1970. Mortality was extremely high during this period, with a peak probability of dying before age 5, $_5q_0$, of 488 per 1,000 live births and an infant mortality rate of 220 in 1966-1970.

Massive interventions were introduced between 1975 and 1983 in three villages. A physician or qualified nursewife was available in the area 24 hours per day. General clinics, as well as prenatal and well-child clinics were held weekly. Women were provided regular gynecological and contraceptive services. To facilitate use of the health services, transportation to and from the clinic was free. Should community members require hospital admission, they were transported to the government hospital. Moreover, traditional midwives were trained to use more hygienic delivery practices. Mortality dropped rapidly. Mortality under age 5 dropped by 75 percent to 110 deaths per 1,000 children in 1982-1983. Infant mortality dropped by 89 percent to only 25 deaths per 1,000 live births. This dramatic decline was achieved by having a physician or a qualified nurse constantly on call. They had a minimal list of essential drugs and means of transportation for referral when necessary.

This case suggests that relatively simple and efficient interventions can bring about a major reduction in mortality in a very short period of time, despite the poor socioeconomic conditions and the low level of education that prevailed throughout the period. It is probably the most striking example of what can be achieved with simple and appropriate interventions.

Niakhar, Senegal, 1962-1989

A rural area of Senegal (Niakhar) has been under demographic surveillance since 1962. During the first period, 1962-1972, mortality was extremely high with an average rate by age 5 of 500 deaths per 1,000 children (Garenne, 1981). There was evidence of mortality decline for all ages and especially for children under 5 years of age since 1962. The decline was not regular. The first major drop in under-5 mortality occurred between 1970 and 1979. Despite the declining trend, annual fluctuations have been considerable, with rates often doubling from one year to the next, most of them being beyond the 95 percent confidence intervals. An attempt to reconstruct the earlier trends in birth and death rates indicated that mortality has declined since at least 1954 and that fertility began to rise at approximately the same time.

A number of interventions were carried out in Niakhar in the late 1970s and through the 1980s. A food supplementation program, which included a growth monitoring component, was carried out between 1972 and 1989. In 1986, a large-scale primary health care program, which included EPI vaccines, oral rehydration therapy, treatment for acute respiratory infections, availability of essential drugs, and medical services, was introduced. Vaccination coverage increased substantially. Measles vaccination coverage increased from 8 percent in 1986 to 80 percent in 1989. The percentage of children receiving the third dose of the DPT vaccine increased from 0 to 56 percent over the same period.

Mortality declined dramatically within three years. Child mortality dropped by 52 percent between 1984-1986 and 1989. During the same period, the infant mortality rate dropped by 41 percent. By 1989, the under-5 mortality rate was 159 deaths per 1,000 children and the infant mortality rate (IMR) was only 69 deaths per 1,000 live births. The neonatal mortality rate was less affected by the project, dropping only 26 percent.

Most of the mortality decline could be attributed to four causes of death that were the target of the interventions: measles, pertussis, diarrhea, and acute respiratory infections. This case study shows that major annual fluctuations are a normal component of child mortality in Africa, that local trends in mortality are far from linear, and above all, that simple selective public health interventions can have a major impact on cause-specific mortality of children in a very short period of time.

HOSPITALS AND HEALTH CENTERS

Table 6-1 presents estimates from the Demographic and Health Surveys (DHS) of the proportion of children with diarrhea, fever, or respiratory problems who received treatment at a medical facility. Basic medical services reach a large proportion of the population of many countries. As a result, the potential effect of these programs is substantial. Despite the large investments in hospitals and health centers, there are very few instances in which the mortality impact of these facilities has been estimated.

Little or no association between child mortality trends in the late 1970s and the availability of health services was reported for Kenya by Blacker et al. (1987), with the exception of a few districts, as discussed in Chapter 7 of the report of the Working Group on Kenya (1993).

The recent DHS in Liberia and Zimbabwe provide an opportunity for a crude test of the effect of health centers. In the Liberia DHS, women reported how long it took them to travel to the nearest clinic. In Zimbabwe, a separate survey was conducted to record the nearest clinic for some of the clusters. Katende (1992) analyzed these data for evidence that proximity to

TABLE 6-1 Proportion of Reported Recent Cases of Diarrhea, Fever, and Cough or Difficulty Breathing Among Children 1-59 Months of Age Taken to a Medical Facility, Selected Countries of Sub-Saharan Africa, 1986-1989

Country	Diarrhea[a]	Fever[b]	Diarrhea and Fever	Cough or Difficulty Breathing[a]	
				Fever	No Fever
Botswana	45.9	90.2	69.1	92.4	81.2
Burundi	38.1	49.9	45.7	45.1	34.8
Ghana	43.1	56.4	48.9	51.5	46.3
Kenya	46.8	55.5	49.7	70.7	56.7
Mali	2.8	2.9	3.3	7.3[c]	3.0[c]
Senegal	19.4	57.6[d]	n.a.	n.a.	n.a.
Togo	25.4	30.8[a]	28.9	36.2[c]	23.9[c]
Uganda	14.8	48.3	18.3	57.6	46.8
Zimbabwe	32.9	n.a.	34.6	58.9	53.5

NOTE: n.a. = not available.

[a]Two weeks preceding survey.
[b]Four weeks preceding survey unless otherwise noted.
[c]Rapid breathing with or without fever.
[d]Malaria during the last cold season.

SOURCE: Boerma et al. (1991:Tables 3.14, 4.2, and 5.2).

a health center is associated with lower infant or child (i.e., ages 1-4 years) mortality. His analysis, which controlled for age, education, socioeconomic status, ethnicity, child immunization status, and water source, did not provide any support for the hypothesis that proximity of health clinics reduce child mortality. The only significant result was for infant mortality in Liberia. Liberian children who live within 30 minutes of a health clinic did appear to have significantly lower infant mortality rates than those who did not. However, this relationship became nonsignificant when several control variables, in particular ethnicity, were included.

We do not consider the results of these analyses to be conclusive. First, cross-sectional data are not suitable for rigorous tests of causality. For example, in areas where a new health clinic opened shortly before the survey, some children may have died before the clinic opened. More significantly, if the government placed clinics in areas where mortality was highest, the cross-sectional results would be biased against finding that clinics reduce mortality. Therefore, it is important to compare the timing of changes in health services to the timing of changes in mortality.

Second, there may not be sufficient variation in accessibility to a clinic to discern a significant effect. In Zimbabwe, particularly, most women included in the survey were within one hour of a clinic. Although the difference between 30 minutes and 60 minutes of travel time might be significant for minor health problems, it might not affect use of the clinic for life-threatening conditions. Because of these problems, it is necessary to rely on studies that examine changing access to health services rather than those providing information at only one point in time.

PRIMARY HEALTH CARE PROGRAMS

Village Health Workers

Greenwood et al. (1990) have measured the effect of the primary health care (PHC) program that began in The Gambia in 1981. The program relied on the work of village health workers (VHWs) and traditional birth attendants (TBAs). The responsibilities of the VHWs included treatment of malaria, diarrhea, and acute respiratory infections, and promotion of improved nutrition and immunization. The VHWs received an initial supply of basic drugs including aspirin, chloroquine, oral penicillin, an antacid, and an anthelmintic. They were to buy replacements with funds obtained through the sale of drugs to their patients. In 1983 the PHC program began in most of the villages in Farafenni district having a population of at least 400. The "non-PHC" villages served as controls. All villages had access to a health center in Farafenni town.

Data on program activities suggest it is unlikely that the VHWs had a large effect on mortality. For example, the VHWs made an average of only one or two visits per child per year. This number was probably too small to have brought about a large mortality decline, especially because there apparently was a perception that the VHWs were not responsible for curative services. Vaccination coverage was already high before the program began (e.g., measles coverage rates of 92 percent in the PHC and 84 percent in the non-PHC villages). Therefore, there was little room for the VHWs to increase vaccination coverage. In addition, the VHWs had only a small impact on the proportion of deceased children who were seen by a doctor before their death. This proportion increased from 48 to 57 percent.

A comparison of the infant and child mortality rates (CMRs) in The Gambia for the year before the start of the program with the rates for the three years after the start show modest, nonsignificant changes. A comparison of the baseline year with the third year after the start of the program does show a significant decline in the IMR. However, the decline in the CMR is still not significant. In addition, there were similar declines in mortality in the non-PHC villages.

The results of the study of PHC in The Gambia are disappointing. However, the sample sizes involved are such that it would be surprising if the differences between PHC and non-PHC villages were significant. If mortality in the PHC villages was actually 20 percent lower than mortality in the non-PHC villages, there would be only a 26 percent chance of finding a difference in infant mortality that was significant at the 5 percent level. There would be only a 30 percent chance of finding such a difference in under-5 mortality. A 20 percent reduction in mortality would be a large reduction, given the differences in level of coverage described above. Therefore, it is not surprising that results fail to show significant differences in mortality.

In addition to the small sample size, it appears that children in non-PHC areas received treatment from VHWs from PHC villages, which would bias the result toward finding no difference in mortality between PHC and non-PHC villages.

Pahou Primary Health Care Project

The Pahou PHC project (Velema et al., 1991) was a field test of an approach to primary health care in Benin. The project covered 16 coastal villages with a population of 13,000 about 30 kilometers from the national capital, Cotonou. The program involved 17 VHWs and vaccination teams that visited each village. The VHWs were trained to visit families with young children and to provide malaria chemoprophylaxis (pyrimethamine) and ORT packets when needed. They were also trained to provide curative services including chloroquine for malaria, sulfadimidine for respiratory infections, mebendazole for parasitic infestations, ORT for diarrhea, and topical aureomycin for eye infections. They also referred patients to the communal health center.

The quality of data collection improved over time, and it is not possible to calculate reliable measures of program impact. In addition, the project did not include a control area. However, Velema et al. (1991) carried out a case-control study to estimate the efficacy of various interventions. The study involved 74 children who died between ages 4 months and 3 years. The deceased children were matched with 230 controls by month of birth, sex, and village of residence. Any interventions received by the controls after the death of the case child were excluded from the analysis.

The intervention associated with the largest reduction of mortality was measles vaccination before 12 months of age. The relative risk for children vaccinated early was 0.36 (95 percent confidence interval (C.I.) 0.16-0.81) compared to unvaccinated children. Measles vaccination after 12 months of age was not associated with any reduction in risk. This curious finding suggests there may be other factors associated with the age at vaccination that contribute to these results. However, the authors state that their results did not change when they included all study variables (among them, apparently, measures of socioeconomic status) in a single logistic regression.

The other EPI vaccinations—DPT, polio, and bacille Calmette-Guérin (BCG)—were not associated with any reduction in mortality. However, the length of the study was so short (34 months) that diphtheria, pertussis, and polio were not prevalent during the study period (Velema et al., 1991). A longer period of observation might have found a greater effect of these vaccinations. Children who received only a single DPT immunization (DPT1) had an elevated risk of death. However, this probably resulted from DPT1 shots given to children who came to the health center for curative services. These sick children were at increased risk of death and were less likely to receive a second DPT.

Estimates of the efficacy of VHW visits applied only to those villages where there was a VHW, thus excluding the two largest villages, which were close to the communal health centers. More than 70 percent of cases and controls were seen by a VHW. Although cases were less likely to have seen a VHW, this difference was not significant. Similarly, the risk of death decreased with the number of contacts with VHWs, but this difference was not significant. However, significantly more controls than cases had been seen by a VHW in the six months preceding the death of the case. Those who had seen a VHW in the past six months had a relative risk of death of 0.33 (95 percent C.I. 0.16-0.69) compared to those who never had contact with a VHW. The number of visits in the most recent six months was also significant.

Unfortunately, the authors do not provide a simple comparison of those

TABLE 6-2 Relative Risk of Death Associated with Timing of VHW Visits in Months Preceding Death, Pahou Primary Health Care Project, Benin, 1986-1987

	Relative Risk	95% C.I.
No visit ≤ 6 months	1.00	
Visits only ≤6 months	0.39	0.16-0.97
≤6 and 7-12 months	0.45	0.16-1.28
≤6, 7-12, and > 12 months	0.30	0.09-0.97
χ^2, 3 df	8.71	

SOURCE: Velema et al. (1991). By permission of Oxford University Press.

who had a visit in the past six months with those who did not. In one test, they examined the relationship between mortality and the number of visits. In another test, they compared those who did not have a visit in the most recent six months with those who had a recent visit, but had not had a visit more than six months ago. The results of the latter analysis are summarized in Table 6-2. The authors concluded that there is evidence of "a linear trend of increasing protection with increasing regularity of contact with the VHW (χ^2 for linear trend: 7.83 on 1 df [degree of freedom])" (Velema et al., 1991:477). However, a reanalysis of the data suggests that the relevant difference is between those who had a recent contact with the VHW (within six months of the age at death of the case) and those who did not.

The Pahou study is an innovative attempt to demonstrate program impact using a case-control design. This approach has the additional advantage of providing some information on the impact of individual interventions. However, the results must be considered tentative because of the likelihood that there are unmeasured differences between families that might affect both mortality and contact with the VHWs. Social class and attitudes toward modern health services are two important sources of variation in both mortality and use of modern services. These factors might be important sources of confounding.

CHILD SURVIVAL AND EXPANDED PROGRAMS ON IMMUNIZATION

Combatting Childhood Communicable Diseases (CCCD) is a program funded by the U.S. Agency for International Development to provide support to child survival programs in Africa. The program provides assistance for increasing vaccination coverage, home-based use of oral rehydration therapy for diarrhea, and presumptive treatment of fevers with chloroquine in malarious areas. Several of the studies quoted in this report were carried out by researchers and program staff associated with CCCD programs (e.g., Cutts, 1988; Taylor et al., 1988; Deming, 1989; Cutts et al., 1990a-b, 1991). In addition, CCCD funded two studies of the effect of child survival activities in areas of two CCCD countries. One was a study of the effect of the national CCCD program on the health services and mortality in Bomi and Grand Cape Mount counties in Liberia. The other examined the effect of the CCCD program in Zaire in the Kingandu area. These studies have the advantage of reporting on the effectiveness of two national programs rather than special demonstration projects.

Evaluation of CCCD in Liberia

Between 1984 and 1988, the CCCD program in Liberia increased coverage with three shots of DPT from 1 to 15 percent and coverage of measles vaccine from 13 to 33 percent among children aged 12 to 23 months. The proportion of pregnancies protected by two injections of tetanus toxoid increased from very low levels to more than 30 percent (Foster et al., 1993).

Becker et al. (1993) reported on the results of two surveys carried out in 1984 and 1988, which recorded mortality rates before and after the start of the program. A comparison of the two years preceding the start of the program with the subsequent two years shows that infant mortality declined by an estimated 24.5 percent (from 240 to 181 death per 1,000 live births). Mortality at ages 1-4 years declined by 28 percent (from 46 to 33 deaths per 1,000). Both changes were significant at the 5 percent level. The study did not include a control area since the program was introduced nationally. However, it is unlikely that declines of this magnitude would have occurred in the absence of the program.

Although it appears that the program reduced mortality overall, the studies did not provide convincing evidence on which components of the program were responsible for the declines. Estimates of the cause of death suggested that mortality due to neonatal tetanus declined by more than 50 percent. Coverage with tetanus toxoid most likely did not increase this much so the decline in tetanus mortality was probably not quite as large. The other cause of death that showed a decline was "fever." However, reported used of antimalarials did not change over the period (Foster et al., 1993). There was no decline in the reporting of measles deaths, nor was there any relationship between the increase in measles coverage by survey cluster and the change in mortality at ages 1-4 years.

The failure of the CCCD study in Liberia to demonstrate declines in causes of death that were targeted by the program is disappointing, but perhaps not surprising. The verbal autopsies employed in the study were taken from questionnaires used in the Philippines. It is not clear to what extent they were valid in Liberia. In addition, the Liberia study used slightly different criteria for diagnosis. For example, in the Philippines, the criteria for diagnosis of nonfatal measles were "age greater than 120 days, rash and fever for more than three days." These criteria had a sensitivity of 98 percent and a specificity of 90 percent (Kalter et al., 1990). Becker et al. (1993) listed their criteria for diagnosis of measles as "presence of skin rash and child over 2 months of age." By dropping fever and not limiting the rash to those lasting at least three days, the specificity of the criteria was probably lower than it was in the Philippines. In addition, dropping the age limit from 4 to 2 months probably led to an exaggeration of measles deaths at ages 1-5 months.

If the sensitivity and specificity of the criteria used in the CCCD study in Liberia were the same as those estimated by Kalter in the Philippines, only about 59 percent of the reported measles deaths in the 1984 were in fact measles.[1] This proportion is termed the "positive predictive value" of the criteria. If the specificity was only 85 percent (because of the less stringent criteria used in Liberia), then only 34 percent of the reported measles deaths were actually due to this cause.

With such low positive predictive values, comparisons of reported measles mortality rates before and after the start of the CCCD program do not provide a powerful test of the hypothesis that the program reduced measles mortality. Because measles immunization coverage increased from 13 to only 33 percent, we might have expected true measles deaths to decline by roughly 20 percent. With a positive predictive value of 59 percent, the expected decline in reported measles deaths would be only 59 percent of 20 percent, or approximately 12 percent, or a decline from about 18 to 16 deaths per 1,000.

There are similar problems with their other reports of causes of death, such as acute respiratory infections. For example, Kalter et al. (1990) estimated that the sensitivity and specificity of "cough for at least 4 days and dyspnoea for at least 1 day" are 59 and 77 percent, respectively. Becker et al. (1993) used the criteria of "cough and trouble breathing for more than 2 days." The positive predictive value for these criteria is probably not high enough to be useful for studying changes in the mortality rate due to respiratory infections.

----

[1]The true proportion of all deaths due to measles can be estimated as $(R + \beta - 1)/(\alpha + \beta - 1)$ where R is the reported proportion due to measles, α is the sensitivity, and β is the specificity.

Evaluation of CCCD in Zaire

The CCCD program in Zaire succeeded in increasing vaccination coverage in the Kingandu area. Measles immunization coverage increased from 22 to 74 percent, and coverage with three doses of DPT increased from 15 to 62 percent (Vernon et al., 1993). Reported use of oral rehydration increased from less than 6 percent to greater than 55 percent per episode. The proportion of pregnancies protected by two injections of tetanus toxoid increased from 14 to 43 percent.

There was an evaluation of the effect of the CCCD program in Zaire in Kingandu (Chahnazarian et al., 1993). The mortality rate among children aged 0 to 5 declined from 41 per 1,000 during the five years preceding the start of the program to 33 during the next five years. This decline was concentrated at ages 1 to 4 years, where mortality declined by 33 percent (95 percent C.I. 22-45 percent). A regression analysis suggested that this decline is more consistent with a program effect than with a steady downward trend, although it is not possible to disentangle the two possibilities statistically.

One approach to determining whether the decline in mortality was due to the program is to examine changes in the reported number of measles cases (Chahnazarian et al., 1993). There was a sharp drop in the annual number of measles cases reported at the local hospital following the start of the program and the increase in vaccination coverage. During 1978-1984, there was an average of 108 measles cases at the hospital each year. After the start of the CCCD program (1985-1989), there was an average of 36 cases per year. Most of these cases occurred during an outbreak in the hospital in 1988. A regression of the mortality rate at ages 6 to 35 months on the reported measles cases for the years 1978-1987 and 1989 shows that variations in the number of reported measles cases explained 67 percent of the variance in mortality. Therefore, the decline in the average annual number of measles cases in the hospital between the preprogram period (1978-1984) and the postprogram period (1985-1989) was associated with an 18 percent decrease in mortality at 6 to 35 months. This estimate probably included some effect from the other program interventions. However, it is likely that the largest share of the effect is attributable to measles immunization.

SUMMARY

It is difficult to believe that the increasing availability of modern health services provided at hospitals, at health centers, and through integrated health programs has not played some role in the long-term decline in infant and child mortality in sub-Saharan Africa. However, there is very little evidence to help us determine whether their contributions have been trivial or substantial. These programs and services are difficult to evaluate because they are based on a set of services rather than a single intervention and are usually introduced slowly over a period of time.

Case histories from Senegal provide some evidence that the declines in mortality were associated with increases in health services. The data from Keneba in The Gambia are more convincing because the health programs were introduced over a period of a few years and were associated with a very rapid decline in mortality.

The evaluations of the CCCD programs are valuable because they are the most recent studies of the effects of national integrated health programs in Africa. Both studies suffer from lack of control areas. In Liberia there were no opportunities for controls, and in Zaire the control area was administratively incorporated into the program area after the start of the study. However, both studies suggested large declines in mortality that were temporally associated with the start of the program.

There is little evidence about the effect of village health workers on mortality. We have not attempted to review all of the literature on the effect of VHW schemes on vaccination coverage, the provision of services by VHWs, and the frequency and timeliness of referrals to clinic. However, the studies reviewed here as well as others (e.g., Nougtara et al., 1989) suggest that VHWs do not necessarily increase utilization of health services.

Many more studies of the effect of primary health care on mortality are needed. Because there is probably great variability in the performance of general health programs, we need more small-scale studies (such as that in The Gambia). Planning small studies will improve the feasibility of completing them. Increasing the number of studies will reveal whether there are any generalizations that can be made about this type of program. Whenever possible, these studies should examine the longer-term effect of programs because it may take several years for them to achieve a level of operation that shows an effect.

7

Conclusions and Recommendations

Health programs in Africa encompass a wide range of medical and public health efforts. Ministries of health often oversee services, such as vaccination programs, maternity services, treatment of chronic psychiatric illnesses, and surgical wards. Given the extremely limited budgets for government expenditures and the pressures for controlling public spending, health sector planners and bilateral or multilateral funding agencies need evidence about whether the programs they support are having the desired effects and guidance on which of these programs and should be expanded.

The circumstantial evidence is clear: The coverage and range of health programs has increased substantially in Africa during the past 20 years, and infant and child mortality rates have declined. However, we found only a few studies that actually measured the effect of any component of a national health program on child mortality in Africa. The vast majority of research comes from studies of defined interventions (e.g., measles vaccination or antimalarial spraying) in small areas. Most of these studies examine the effects of a single intervention, and many are closer to carefully controlled clinical trials than they are to evaluations of large-scale programs. Therefore, we cannot make strong statements about the overall effectiveness of health programs in Africa. However, we can conclude that most national health programs include interventions that have been shown to reduce mortality in small test programs.

Our first and most important finding is that many of the central elements of most national health programs in Africa have never been evaluated in terms of their likely impact on mortality. In some cases, the nature of the programs and of the interventions precludes direct measurement of effectiveness in reducing mortality. However, there are many types of programs that could be evaluated but have not been studied or have been studied only in small-scale trials. In particular, there are very few studies of the effects of health centers and integrated programs on mortality, and no studies that attempt to estimate the effectiveness of hospitals in reducing population levels of mortality.

Given this conclusion, most of the review of the evidence—and, therefore, most of the conclusions below—concern interventions aimed at individual diseases. We will summarize here our findings about the four most common causes of death among children in Africa: measles, diarrhea, malaria, and acute respiratory infections.

DISEASE- AND INTERVENTION-SPECIFIC CONCLUSIONS

Measles

Vaccination programs currently provide measles vaccination to about half of all children in the region. The protective effects of measles vaccination are well documented in several studies in coastal areas of West Africa and one study in Zaire. In these locales, vaccination was responsible for substantial declines in mortality. There is evidence from several other areas that vaccination has reduced the incidence of measles. However, wide variations in vaccine efficacy (often associated with cold chain failures) and substantial differences in the epidemiology of the disease (e.g., frequency of epidemics, proportion secondary cases) make it difficult to estimate the impact of measles vaccination in Africa.

Vaccination is not likely to eliminate measles cases in Africa in the near future. Therefore, expanded case management should be considered as a supplemental strategy to lower the case-fatality rates in serious cases.

Diarrheal Diseases

Diarrheal diseases are among the leading causes of death of infants and children in sub-Saharan Africa, as they are throughout the developing world. They also reduce the health of children by imposing a high burden of morbidity and by contributing substantially to malnutrition. The primary intervention for control of diarrheal disease mortality in the past decade has been management of acute dehydrating diarrhea by using oral rehydration therapy (ORT) and continued feeding. This approach to case management has proven efficacious in clinical settings outside of Africa and is likely to prevent mortality in community-wide programs, but the effects in community-based programs have not been well documented in Africa. To achieve the maximum benefit from this intervention in sub-Saharan Africa, it would be necessary to increase coverage beyond the currently estimated 36 percent of episodes treated, and to improve both the targeting of treatment and the quality of the treatment given. Furthermore, because acute dehydrating illnesses may be responsible for half or less of diarrhea-associated mortality, a more comprehensive approach to case management will also be needed to reduce the mortality due to dysentery and persistent diarrhea, often associated with malnutrition.

Malaria

Presumptive treatment of fever with chloroquine is standard practice in many parts of Africa. It is not only the practice in health centers; presumptive treatment is practiced in many homes before or instead of attending a health center. There are no studies demonstrating that presumptive treatment actually reduces childhood mortality. Although studies demonstrate the effect of treatment of malaria with chloroquine on the progression of the disease, there are no studies that test the basic assumption that reducing case severity will in the long run reduce mortality.

It may not be possible to design studies to compare the effectiveness of presumptive treatment with no treatment of fevers. It would be unethical to remove this treatment from a control population that already relies on chloroquine, and it might not be possible to find endemic or holoendemic areas where presumptive treatment is not already practiced. However, it would be possible to test the effect of increasing the proportion of cases treated presumptively or the effect of improving dosages or promptness of treatment. The two studies designed to do so failed to bring about sizable changes in the frequency of treatment.

The effectiveness of presumptive treatment with chloroquine is also uncertain because of increases in the prevalence of chloroquine resistance. Although the mere presence of resistant strains does not mean that chloroquine is totally useless, it does reduce the level of effectiveness. As long as chloroquine was effective, the arguments for presumptive treatment were persuasive. However, the reduced efficacy of chloroquine and the lack of equally safe, low-cost alternative drugs introduce additional uncertainty into the estimation of effectiveness.

Home-based use of chloroquine and other drugs for presumptive treatment of fevers presents problems for research on the effectiveness of other strategies for reducing mortality due to malaria. Researchers cannot assume that the level of treatment or chemoprophylaxis is minimal in designated control areas or at the time of baseline surveys in intervention areas. It is necessary to document the frequency and adequacy of treatment (home based and at clinics, presumptive and diagnosed). Without documentation of the level of treatment in control areas or baseline comparisons of program and control areas, study results cannot be extrapolated to areas in which the baseline conditions may be quite different.

The evidence substantiating the use of chemoprophylaxis among pregnant women is not very strong. Although there are numerous studies demonstrating beneficial effects of prophylaxis on intermediate outcomes such as birthweight, there is little direct evidence that prophylaxis actually increases child survival.

The use of insecticide-impregnated bed nets has been demonstrated to reduce mortality in one area of sub-Saharan Africa with high levels of seasonal malaria. There is a need for studies of acceptability and efficacy in populations with other patterns, such as areas of high endemicity and areas of infrequent epidemics.

Acute Respiratory Infections

Acute respiratory infections (ARIs), particularly pneumonia, are also a major cause of childhood mortality in sub-Saharan Africa. Although their importance has been recognized for some time, it is only recently that a control program strategy has been shown to be effective. This strategy uses a presumptive diagnostic algorithm of pneumonia based principally on respiratory rate and recognition of chest indrawing; treatment is given with antibiotics. In community-based intervention trials in a variety of settings, this strategy has been shown to reduce under-5 mortality by approximately 25 percent. In the only trial in sub-Saharan Africa, the probability of dying by age 5 was reduced by 39 per 1,000. Clearly, some antibiotic treatment of suspected pneumonia is currently occurring in Africa, but systematic programs to improve diagnosis and provide correct therapy are just beginning. Although it is too soon to determine an effect on child mortality of ARI treatment programs, there would seem to be the potential for substantial mortality reduction if the case-management strategy can be fully implemented.

GENERAL OBSERVATIONS ABOUT THE EVALUATION OF HEALTH PROGRAMS IN AFRICA

Given the wide range of disease environments in Africa, a worrying number of the best studies of the efficacy of basic interventions have been carried out in a very narrow range of ecological and cultural settings. In particular, a substantial proportion of the studies have been carried out in small areas of Senegal and The Gambia. The area of Senegal that has been studied by researchers from the Institut Français de Recherche Scientifique pour le Développement en Coopération (ORSTOM), and the area of The Gambia that has been studied by researchers from the Medical Research Council of the United Kingdom, are within approximately 60 miles of each other in very similar ecological and cultural environments. Good research is being done in other areas of Africa. However, there is a desperate need for more research on the effectiveness of integrated programs and individual interventions in a wider range of environments. The high volume of excellent research from Senegal and The Gambia is evidence that long-term studies in defined populations are an effective means of studying health interventions.

In addition to disease- and intervention-specific conclusions and recommendations, there are a number of general observations related to the state of health programs and research in sub-Saharan Africa.

1. **Declines in infant and child mortality rates should remain the primary indicator of the effectiveness of child health interventions in Africa.** There are other useful indicators of the success of some specific health interventions, such as improved nutritional status and lower prevalence of chronic morbidity. However, the primary goal of most health programs in Africa must be the reduction of mortality. In addition, many of the interventions aimed at reducing mortality are also associated with reductions in morbidity.

That having been said, it is not necessary to measure the change in mortality associated with every program. Once we have shown that an intervention reduces mortality when implemented properly, we can evaluate programs using coverage and promptness of services and compliance with program protocols.

2. **The goals stated for many programs suggest that program planners often have unrealistic expectations about the feasibility of measuring mortality changes associated with some kinds of interventions.** There is large variation in the rapidity with which interventions can reduce mortality. It is feasible to measure the effects only of those interventions that can achieve large reductions in mortality quickly. Evaluation of interventions that reduce mortality by only a modest amount (e.g., less than 10 percent) requires very large sample sizes to achieve precise measurements of mortality. However, the larger the sample size, the more difficult it is to ensure precise measurements. For national programs, it may not be possible to measure the effect of programs that reduce mortality in an age group by less than 20 per 1,000.

Similarly, it may not be possible to demonstrate that a program reduced mortality if the mortality decline occurred over several years. The slower the decline, the longer must data collection continue and the greater is the expense. A long, slow decline also makes it difficult to demonstrate that the change was caused by the program rather than by other changes in the population.

It is useful to consider three types of programs:

• Programs that are relatively easy to study because they have a dramatic effect on mortality: Included here are programs that can cause a quick, dramatic reduction in mortality, perhaps limited to one age group. In some cases, it is possible to document the effectiveness of these programs in large populations. Examples are programs that include measles vaccination and mass immunization of women of childbearing age with tetanus toxoid. Regular distribution of vitamin A may also belong in this group. Although evaluations of these programs can demonstrate short-term effects on mortality, studies of long-term, sustained effectiveness generally will have to rely on intermediate measures such as vaccine efficacy and surveillance studies of incidence.

• Programs whose effectiveness in reducing mortality can be measured only in small-scale studies: This group includes programs that have a more modest potential for reducing mortality or that reduce mortality at a slower rate. We can strengthen these studies by comparing survival rates for those who received the intervention and those who did not. Examples include programs for treatment of ARI and immunization of pregnant women with tetanus toxoid. Once the effectiveness of these programs has been demonstrated in small-scale studies, larger programs can be evaluated by using intermediate measures such as coverage rates, efficacy, and incidence rates.

• Programs for which direct measurement of effect on mortality is not feasible: This group includes programs that require an expansion of infrastructure, establishing a referral structure, a large change in staff duties, or changes in health-seeking behavior or treatment of disease by the population. These programs can take so long to be implemented fully that it is very difficult, if not impossible, to document their effects in populations. In addition, it is often difficult to document a single starting point for these programs or to measure changes in the level of program activity. This category includes programs to reduce the incidence of low birthweight and prematurity. In general, we can only estimate the effectiveness of these programs by using studies of intermediate output measures (e.g., coverage rates and changes in the incidence of low birthweight) combined with studies that demonstrate the association of these intermediate variables with excess mortality.

Misunderstandings about the nature of program effect can lead to unrealistic expectations for measurable impact. For example, many discussions of the potential of home-based ORT programs imply that they can achieve quick, dramatic reductions in mortality. In fact, such programs belong in the second or even third group because of the time required to implement them and to change behaviors. Similarly, programs that provide tetanus toxoid can achieve large reductions in some populations if coverage increases rapidly. However, programs that provide injections through antenatal care may not achieve a quick increase in coverage in populations where prenatal care is low. The foregoing does not mean that we should invest only in programs that have quick effects. However, we should ensure that the measures used to evaluate these programs are firmly linked to real effects.

3. **The trend toward stating program goals in terms of reduction in cause-specific mortality may be setting unrealistic expectations for evaluation.** Measuring cause-specific mortality rates is very difficult in Africa. Even carefully performed verbal autopsies using locally validated methods can only provide estimates of the distribution of deaths by the most common immediate causes. Assigning associated or underlying causes exceeds the capabilities of large studies and national systems. In general, it is not possible to measure cause of death precisely enough for the evaluation of large-scale programs. However, it is important to produce better national and subnational estimates of the relative importance of major causes of death and to develop systems for monitoring long-term trends in the cause-of-death structure. The verbal autopsy components of the Demographic and Health Surveys and other surveys should begin to give some ideas of the mortality profiles of infants and children in the general population.

4. **More emphasis should be given to age-specific mortality rates in stating program goals.** It is far easier to measure achievement of goals for reduction of neonatal, postneonatal, or second-year mortality, for example, than goals for reducing disease-specific mortality. It is often possible to identify age (or age-sex) groups that should benefit most from a program.

5. **There is a need for more evaluations of various packages of interventions.** For example, there may soon be a need to evaluate the combination of vaccination programs and vitamin A distribution. The purpose of these evaluations should be to measure the total impact of the package. It is rarely possible to determine which elements of a package are responsible for the largest share of the effect. The synergies between diseases make it as difficult to estimate the joint effect of two interventions from separate evaluations as it is to disentangle their separate effects when they are studied in combination. Because the impact of various packages can differ greatly across disease environments, we should evaluate these packages in several types of populations.

6. **More empirical evaluation of program effects are needed in order to test predictions from models.** Although we have data on many components of these models, there are no direct tests of the effects of the recommended practices. Examples include the training of traditional birth attendants and several of the common recommendations on malaria. We are

not suggesting that programs stop training traditional birth attendants or change their recommendations on malaria. Whenever possible, the conclusions from simplified biological models should be tested in studies that actually measure the effectiveness of the proposed intervention in reducing mortality.

7. **There is a need for more long-term studies that include regular collection of vital statistics and routine surveys of service utilization and quality of care.** These studies require long-term commitments of funds and personnel. However, their potential is apparent from the number of important studies carried out in Senegal and The Gambia. Without these study areas, we would know much less about such diseases as measles and malaria, and the potential effect of interventions to combat them. We need similar types of study areas in other parts of Africa.

Similarly, on-going data collection programs, such as the Demographic and Health Survey program, should continue gathering information on health services and conditions. These surveys can contribute to the knowledge base of long-term health and population changes in sub-Saharan Africa.

8. **Evaluation studies should include detailed measurement of both the coverage and the promptness of services, as well as compliance with program protocols.** We cannot adequately evaluate measurements of mortality change associated with programs unless we also have data on the program activities.

During the last 10 years there has been a great deal of attention paid to the health needs of Africa. Many programs have been started or expanded, and many new approaches have been tested in clinical trials and small study areas. Despite this increased effort, we know very little about the effects of single interventions in large-scale national programs or the overall effectiveness of integrated health programs. There are also many parts of the continent where we know very little about the effect of programs or even the efficacy of treatments. The need for program evaluations will increase as the recommended combinations of interventions become more elaborate. In particular, if we begin to consider adding large-scale intervention against acute respiratory infections or vitamin A supplementation to the existing vaccination and diarrhea control programs, it will be increasingly difficult to evaluate programs without direct measurements of their effect. As the size and the complexity of programs increase, so will the need for more elaborate systems to evaluate and monitor their effectiveness, and to set new priorities.

Appendix A

Case Studies of Child Mortality

Data from national systems of vital statistics are incomplete and usually unpublished. Therefore, we have to rely on specific population-based surveys, a special analysis of vital registration data for small areas, or hospital records to estimate the structure of the causes of death among infants and children in sub-Saharan Africa.

This appendix includes summaries of 9 case studies that provide some data on the causes of death among infants and children. These studies are of very uneven quality and differ in the amount of details they provide. The data are drawn from three types of sources: vital statistics, hospital records, and population surveillance systems. Each of these sources has its limitations. Vital registration systems may record a large number of deaths, but if deaths are unattended or not certified by a physician, the reported cause of death may well be incorrect. Hospital data may be more accurate in determining the cause, but they are subject to a selection bias. Population surveillance systems generally have excellent coverage and consistent diagnosis of cause of death, but they are based on small populations and generally limited to a few years. Their results may therefore produce a good picture of a fairly small area and population, but it may be difficult to make generalizations based upon their findings. Where it is possible, these results also include the percentages of death attributed to other and undetermined causes.

SIERRA LEONE (WESTERN AREA)

Infant and child mortality in Sierra Leone is among the highest in the world, with the infant mortality rate (IMR) between 1980 and 1985 estimated at 166 per 1,000 live births (United Nations, 1991). Kandeh (1986) conducted an analysis of the causes of infant and childhood deaths in the Western Area of the country where the main hospitals for mothers and children are located.

Of the 3,783 infant deaths recorded in the vital registration system of the Western Area between 1969 and 1971, only 1,772 (47 percent) were medically certified. Of these deaths, 33 percent (582) occurred during the first week of life, 27 percent (483) between the second and fourth weeks, and the remaining 40 percent (707) during the second through eleventh months. As shown in Table A-1, neonatal mortality was dominated by tetanus (41 percent), which was also the leading cause of death in infancy. This cause was followed by "anoxic and hypoxic conditions," which accounted for 18 percent of neonatal deaths. Both conditions are closely associated with poor care of the delivery and of the newborn child. Other important causes of neonatal death were pneumonia and other acute respiratory infections (ARIs) (6 percent), birth infection (5 percent), congenital anomaly (3 percent), and septicemia (1 percent). Postneonatal mortality was due primarily to pneumonia (30 percent) and other ARIs (5 percent), diarrhea (21 percent), measles (9 percent), and malaria (6 percent). Malnutrition per se was not coded, but may be included among avitaminosis (3 percent) and anemia (4 percent), although this last category probably reflects malaria mortality as well.

Medically certified deaths of children between ages 1 and 4 years were attributed to measles (22 percent), pneumonia (22 percent), diarrhea (13 percent), avitaminosis (10 percent), anemia (10 percent), malaria (4 percent), tuberculosis (3 percent), meningitis (2 percent), accidents (1 percent), dysentery (1 percent), and other causes (10 percent).

This study covered a large population and included both an urban and a rural area. The results are similar to other studies (see Table 2-3 for comparison). However, a few features limit the comparability with other studies: Severe malnutrition was not coded as a cause of death; pertussis was either neglected or included in the "other ARI" category; malaria played a smaller role than elsewhere, which may be due to reporting biases or to the local environment; diarrhea seemed to have been underestimated; and some categories were unconventional (such as anoxic and hypoxic conditions).

TABLE A-1 Ranking of Major Underlying Causes of Death in Sierra Leone (western area) by Age Group, 1969-1979

Rank	Neonatal (N = 1,065), 1969-1971		Postneonatal (N = 732), 1969-1971		Children, Aged 1-4 (N = 924), 1974-1976	
	Cause of Death	Percentage	Cause of Death	Percentage	Cause of Death	Percentage
1	Tetanus	41.1	Pneumonia	30.4	Measles	22.3
2	Anoxic/hypoxic	18.3	Diarrhea	21.2	Pneumonia	22.2
3	Pneumonia	5.1	Measles	9.1	Diarrhea	13.1
4	Birth infection	4.6	Malaria	6.0	Avitaminosis	10.3
5	Congenital anomalies	3.3	Other ARI	5.0	Anemia	9.7
6	Diarrhea	1.6	Anemia	4.2	Malaria	4.6
7	Septicemia	1.4	Avitaminosis	2.9	Tuberculosis	3.1
8			Tetanus	2.4	Meningitis	2.2
9			Septicemia	1.6	Accidents	1.3
10			Congenital anomalies	0.9	Dysentery	0.8

SOURCE: Kandeh (1986).

MACHAKOS, KENYA

The Machakos area of Kenya (1975-1978) had a much lower mortality rate than other areas of Africa, which may imply a different cause-of-death structure. Data were collected in this rural area between 1975 and 1978. Omondi-Odhiambo et al. (1990) report that in the neonatal period, after asphyxia and prematurity, which accounted for almost half of the deaths, the leading cause of death was ARI, which was associated with 18 percent. The cause of 15 percent of the neonatal deaths was unknown. During the postneonatal period, the leading causes were intestinal infections and pneumonia (40 and 28 percent, respectively), followed by measles (14 percent). Only 7 percent were reported as unknown cause. Among children ages 1 to 4 years, measles was responsible for 32 percent of all deaths. Nutritional deficiencies were the cause of 17 percent of all child deaths. Pneumonia and diarrhea were listed as causing 13 and 14 percent of deaths, respectively. Pneumonia and diarrhea were more important among infants than among children aged 1-4 years, whereas measles and malnutrition were more often the causes of death of children; 4 percent were of unknown cause.

NATIONAL ESTIMATES FOR KENYA

Ewbank et al. (1986) used data from 1976 to 1987 on hospital inpatient deaths, registered deaths by district, and results of available epidemiologic data (including the Machakos study) to estimate the cause-of-death structure for Kenya. They attempted to adjust for the selectivity of hospital deaths and for the fact that both the coverage of registered deaths and the distribution of deaths by cause differ among districts.

Their estimates of the number of deaths by cause for children under age five are given in Table A-2. In addition, they estimated that there were about 10,900 deaths at all ages due to malaria. Because a large proportion

TABLE A-2 Under-5 Cause-of-Death Structure of Kenya

Cause of Death	Estimated Number of Deaths	Percent
Respiratory	26,600	50.0
Measles	14,600	27.5
Diarrhea	9,300	17.5
Neonatal tetanus	2,200	4.2
Pertussis	400	0.8
Total	53,100	100.0

SOURCE: Ewbank et al. (1986).

of malaria deaths occur to children under age 5, malaria would rank about fourth on this list.

DAKAR AND SAINT-LOUIS, SENEGAL

Cantrelle et al. (1986) studied vital registration data from the cities of Dakar and Saint-Louis, between 1973 and 1980. The quality of the data on causes of death was to a large extent determined by the place of death. When the death occurred in a health unit, as was the case for 68 percent of the deaths in Dakar and 58 percent in Saint-Louis, the cause of death was more precise because it was generally established by a physician. When the death occurred at home, a public official was left to determine the cause.

In Dakar, congenital disorders and perinatal diseases were the cause of 25 percent of all infant deaths; in Saint-Louis, these causes were responsible for 33 percent of all infant deaths. The percentages varied over the eight-year period, with a range of 19 to 30 percent observed in Dakar and 23 to 48 percent in Saint-Louis. In Dakar, the second leading cause of infant mortality was diarrhea, accounting for 11.6 percent of deaths. In Saint-Louis, malnutrition and dehydration (combined into one category) were listed as the second leading cause of infant death, with 17 percent. Measles was the third leading cause in both cities, accounting for 10 percent in Dakar and 7 percent in Saint-Louis. Of infant deaths in Dakar, 6 percent were attributed to malnutrition and dehydration, followed by bronchopulmonary disorders (6 percent). Diarrhea, the fourth leading cause of infant mortality in Saint-Louis, was responsible for 5 percent of the deaths, followed by bronchopulmonary disorders (5 percent). The remaining deaths were attributable to other causes or could not be determined.

For children, the leading cause of deaths in both cities was measles. In Dakar, measles was listed as the cause of 28 percent of the deaths, whereas in Saint-Louis, it was responsible for 21 percent. Diarrheal and intestinal diseases were the second leading cause of death in Dakar (12 percent), and the third major cause in Saint-Louis (10 percent). Malnutrition and dehydration were the second major cause of child death in Saint-Louis, accounting for 18 percent. Malaria was also a major cause of death in Saint-Louis, with 9 percent, whereas in Dakar, it was much less important, with only 2 percent. On the other hand, bronchopulmonary disorders accounted for 9 percent of the child deaths in Dakar, but only 4 percent in Saint-Louis.

Cantrelle et al. (1986) pointed out that ecological conditions should be considered when examining trends. A major drought in Saint-Louis in 1972 and 1973 probably reduced food production, thus contributing to the high percentage of deaths from malnutrition and dehydration. Moreover, heavy rainfall in Saint-Louis during 1975 corresponded to an increase in deaths from malaria, a cause that was relatively unimportant in Dakar. With respect to infant mortality, they indicated that with the exception of measles, other major causes of death were often associated with the consequences of low rainfall and drought, such as low crop production and reduced purchasing power.

NIAKHAR, SENEGAL

Garenne and Fontaine (1990) analyzed 808 verbal autopsies recorded by a demographic surveillance system in Niakhar, a rural area of Senegal. All deaths of all ages occurring in 30 villages were studied by using a comprehensive questionnaire. Results for children below age 5 for the years 1983-1989 are shown in Table A-3 (M. Garenne, personal communication, 1992).

Two causes accounted for more than half of all neonatal deaths: neonatal tetanus and low birthweight. The few cases of malnutrition involved newborns who were improperly nourished because their mothers died shortly after delivery. For postneonatal mortality, diarrhea and acute respiratory infections accounted for half of all deaths. Pertussis accounted for more deaths than measles, because this disease strikes soon after birth, whereas cases of measles are extremely rare before 4 months of age.

For children aged 1-4 years, diarrhea was still the most common cause of death. Malaria and acute malnutrition were more important than ARI. Measles preceded pertussis and cholera, which was very rare among infants. Hepatitis and tuberculosis were probably underestimated, because of the less typical symptoms that are harder to identify by using verbal autopsies. Deaths due to typhoid and congenital syphilis were never diagnosed, but do exist in the study area.

In this study, malnutrition included acute malnutrition (kwashiorkor and marasmus) and three cases of anemia, which may have been caused by malaria. An independent study of risk factors showed that two-thirds of the deaths outside the neonatal period were attributable to poor nutritional status. The diarrhea category for postneonates included acute watery diarrhea (16 percent), persistent diarrhea (12 percent), and dysentery (2 percent); and for children 1-4, acute watery diarrhea (9 percent), persistent diarrhea (16 percent), and dysentery (3 percent).

BAMAKO, MALI

A study of the vital statistics collected between 1974 and 1985 in Bamako, Mali, provides information on cause-of-death structure (Fargues and Nassour, 1988). Registration of deaths is virtually complete in Bamako because a death certificate from the government is needed for burial. If death occurs in a hospital, the cause of death is noted by the attending physician or

TABLE A-3 Ranking of Major Underlying Causes of Death in Niakhar, Senegal, 1983-1989, by Age Group

Rank	Neonatal (N = 407)		Postneonatal (N = 461)		Children Aged 1-4 (N = 1,015)	
	Cause of Death	Percentage	Cause of Death	Percentage	Cause of Death	Percentage
1	Tetanus	39.1	Diarrhea	29.9	Diarrhea	27.4
2	Low birth weight	28.0	ARI	19.5	Malaria	12.0
3	Pneumonia	4.9	Malaria	6.9	Malnutrition	8.5
4	Birth trauma	2.2	Pertussis	6.1	ARI	8.3
5	Birth defect	1.7	Malnutrition	5.4	Measles	8.0
6	Diarrhea	1.0	Measles	3.7	Pertussis	4.2
7	Malnutrition	0.5	Meningitis	2.7	Cholera	3.7
8			Septicemia	1.3	Meningitis	2.0
9			Varicella	1.0	Varicella	0.5
10					Septicemia	0.4
11					Epilepsy	0.4
12					Hepatitis	0.3
13					Tuberculosis	0.3

SOURCE: M. Garenne, personal communication (1992).

nurse. However, for a death that occurs at home, the certificate may not accurately reflect the true cause of death. Some causes of death such as measles are easily recognizable to individuals reporting the death, but other causes such as dehydration may be reported incorrectly as diarrhea. Similarly, many people are aware of fever as a symptom of malaria and report deaths as being caused by malaria when a high fever is present.

The leading causes of infant mortality were conditions related to the perinatal period (prematurity), which accounted for 24 percent of the deaths. Following that, 12 percent were attributed to malaria, whereas measles was responsible for 10 percent. The fourth leading cause was intestinal infection, accounting for 9 percent. The other major causes of death were meningitis (4 percent), malnutrition (4 percent), dehydration (4 percent), and pneumonia (3 percent). The remaining causes of death either accounted for less than 1 percent of the total, and approximately 28 percent were classified as "other."

Among children of ages 1 to 5, measles was reported as the cause of 34 percent of deaths, followed by malaria with 16 percent. In this group, 12 percent was attributed to malnutrition, whereas intestinal infection accounted for 8 percent. Pneumonia and dehydration each accounted for 3 percent of the deaths; anemia and meningitis, 1 percent each. Approximately 20 percent of deaths to children ages 1 to 5 years were attributed to other causes.

MALUMFASHI, NIGERIA

Data collected by Tomkins et al. (1991) between 1977 and 1978 in the Malumfashi area of Nigeria yielded basic cause of death information. During this period, 111 infants died, resulting in an infant mortality rate of 88 deaths per 1,000 live births. Among these infants, 12 percent were reported to have died of measles, 23 percent of pyrexia, and 13 percent of diarrhea. Among children ages 1 to 4, a similar pattern was observed. With a child mortality rate of 34 deaths per 1,000 (137 deaths), 12 percent of the deaths were ascribed to measles, 24 percent to pyrexia, and 17 percent to diarrhea.

FOUR PROVINCES OF SUDAN

Verbal autopsies provide information on the deaths of infants and children in a study in Greater Khartoum and the Blue Nile, Kassala, and Kordofan provinces of the Sudan between 1974 and 1976 (Sudanese Ministry of Health and World Health Organization, 1981). It appears that infant mortality was probably underreported. Among infants, 48 percent of the deaths were attributed to diarrhea and 12 percent to fevers. Measles was responsible for 11 percent of infant deaths, followed by pneumonia (9 percent), malaria (5 percent), and asphyxia (4 percent). The remaining 11 percent of deaths were attributed to other and undetermined causes. The leading causes of death among children were diarrhea (46 percent), measles (18 percent), malaria (7 percent), pneumonia (6 percent), and fever (6 percent); 18 percent were attributed to other and undetermined causes.

KASONGO, ZAIRE

The Kasongo study was conducted in Zaire between 1974 and 1977 (van Lerberghe, 1989). The survey gathered information on 229 deaths of children under age 5, and deaths were classified into five groups: rash, respiratory disease, diarrheal disease, other diseases, and unknown. Those classified as rashes were attributed to measles if the child had a rash that started less than 30 days before the death. Respiratory deaths included those in which the mother attributed the death to a respiratory illness (cough, dyspnea, or whooping cough), dyspnea or cough were reported at death, or respiratory illness was reported between the preceding visit and death. Deaths were ascribed to diarrhea when they were attributed to diarrhea by the mother or when there was mention of diarrhea at death if there was no association with rash, respiratory illness, or any other specific cause of death.

Among the deaths of infants under 5 months of age, 40 percent were of unknown origin and 30 percent were classified as "other" causes. Respiratory illnesses were the leading identifiable cause, representing about 20 percent of all deaths. Diarrhea was reported as the cause of about 7 percent, and rash about 3 percent.

Among older children, rash (measles) was the leading cause of death: approximately 45 percent of the deaths among children 6 to 11 months, and 75 percent among children 12 to 17 months. In the groups aged 18 to 59 months, rashes were the largest single cause, ranging from about 60 to 35 percent, respectively. Respiratory illnesses and diarrhea each caused about 20 percent of the deaths among infants between 6 and 11 months, and only about 5 percent each in the age group 12 to 17 months. Diarrheal diseases accounted for about 10 percent of the deaths between ages 18 and 47 months, but were not cited as the cause of death in the group aged 48 to 59 months. Respiratory illnesses were reported to be the cause of about 20 percent of the deaths among children 24-35 months and 48-59 months. However, respiratory illnesses were not listed as the cause of any deaths among children 36-47 months. Among children 6 to 59 months, unknown causes of death ranged from approximately 2 to 15 percent of the total of registered deaths.

Appendix B

Demographic and Health Survey (DHS) Reports

The following references are included in citations of DHS reports:

Agounké, A., M. Assogba, and K. Anipah
  1989   *Enquête Démographique et de Santé au Togo 1988.* Lomé, Togo: Unité de Recherche Démographique, Direction de la Statistique, Direction Générale de la Santé; Columbia, Md.: Institute for Resource Development/Macro Systems, Inc.

Chieh-Johnson, D., A.R. Cross, A.A. Way, and J.M. Sullivan
  1988   *Liberia Demographic and Health Survey 1986.* Monrovia, Liberia: Bureau of Statistics, Ministry of Planning and Economic Affairs; Columbia, Md.: Institute for Resource Development/Westinghouse.

Ghanaian Statistical Service and Institute for Resource Development
  1989   *Ghana Demographic and Health Survey 1988.* Accra, Ghana: Ghana Statistical Services; Columbia, Md.: Institute for Resource Development/Macro Systems, Inc.

Kaijuka, E.M., E.Z.A. Kaija, A.R. Cross, and E. Loaiza
  1989   *Uganda Demographic and Health Survey 1988/1989.* Entebbe, Uganda: Ministry of Health; Columbia, Md.: Institute for Resource Development/Macro Systems, Inc.

Kenyan National Council for Population and Development and Institute for Resource Development
  1989   *Kenya Demographic and Health Survey 1989.* Nairobi, Kenya: National Council for Population and Development; Columbia, Md.: Institute for Resource Development/Macro Systems, Inc.

Lesetedi, L.T., G.D. Mompati, P. Khulumani, G.N. Lesetedi, N. Rutenberg
  1989   *Botswana Family Health Survey II.* Gaborone, Botswana: Central Statistics Office (Ministry of Finance and Development Planning) and Family Health Division

(Ministry of Health); Columbia, Md.: Institute for Resource Development/ Macro Systems, Inc.

Ndiaye, S., I. Sarr, and M. Ayad

    1988   *Enquête Démographique et de Santé au Sénégal 1986.* Dakar, Senegal: Ministère de l'Economie et de Finances; Columbia, Md.: Institute for Resource Development/Westinghouse.

Nigerian Federal Office of Statistics and Institute for Resource Development

    1992   *Nigeria Demographic and Health Survey 1990.* Lagos, Nigeria: Federal Office of Statistics; Columbia, Md.: Institute for Resource Development/Macro International, Inc.

Segamba, L., V. Ndikumasabo, C. Makinson, and M. Ayad

    1988   *Enquête Démographique et de Santé au Burundi.* Gitega, Burundi: Ministère de l'Intérieur; Columbia, Md.: Institute for Resource Development/Westinghouse.

Traore, B., M. Konate, and C. Stanton

    1989   *Enquête Démographique et de Santé au Mali 1987.* Bamako, Mali: Centre d'Etudes et de Recherches sur la Population pour le Développement; Columbia, Md.: Institute for Resource Development/Westinghouse.

University of Zambia, Central Statistical Office, and Institute for Resource Development

    1992   *Zambia Demographic and Health Survey 1992 (Preliminary Report).* Lusaka, Zambia: University of Zambia and Central Statistical Office; Columbia, Md.: Institute for Resource Development/Macro International, Inc.

Zimbabwe Central Statistical Office and Institute for Resource Development

    1989   *Zimbabwe Demographic and Health Survey 1988.* Harare, Zimbabwe: Central Statistical Office; Columbia, Md.: Institute for Resource Development/Macro Systems, Inc.

References

Aaby, P.
  1988   *Malnourished or Overinfected: An Analysis of the Determinants of Acute Measles Mortality.* Copenhagen: Laegeforeningens Forlag.
  1992   Overcrowding and intensive exposure: Major determinants of variations in measles mortality in Africa. Pp. 317-348 in E. van de Walle, G. Pison, and M.D. Sala-Diakanda, eds., *Mortality and Society in Sub-Saharan Africa.* New York: Oxford University Press.
Aaby, P., and J. Leeuwenberg
  1990   Patterns of transmission and severity of measles infection: A reanalysis of data from the Machakos area, Kenya. *Journal of Infectious Diseases* 161:171-174.
Aaby, P., J. Bukh, I.M. Lisse, A.J. Smits, J. Gomes, M.A. Fernandes, F. Indi, and M. Soares
  1984a   Determinants of measles mortality in a rural area of Guinea-Bissau: Crowding, age, and malnutrition. *Journal of Tropical Pediatrics* 30:164-168.
Aaby, P., J. Bukh, I.M. Lisse, and A.J. Smits
  1984b   Measles vaccination and reduction in child mortality: A community study from Guinea-Bissau. *Journal of Infectious Diseases* 8:13-21.
  1984c   Overcrowding and intensive exposure as determinants of measles mortality. *American Journal of Epidemiology* 120(1):49-63.
Aaby, P., J. Bukh, J. Leerhoy, I.M. Lisse, C.H. Mordhorst, and I.R. Pedersen
  1986   Vaccinated children get milder measles infection: A community study from Guinea-Bissau. *Journal of Infectious Diseases* 154(5):858-863.
Aaby, P., J. Bukh, I.M. Lisse, and M.C. da Silva
  1988a   Decline in measles mortality: Nutrition, age at infection, or exposure? *British Medical Journal* 296:1225-1228.
Aaby, P., T.G. Jensen, H.L. Hansen, and H. Kristiansen
  1988b   Trial of high-dose Edmonston-Zagreb measles vaccine in Guinea-Bissau: Protective efficacy. *Lancet* (ii):809-811.

166

Aaby, P., I.R. Pedersen, K. Knudsen, M.C. da Silva, C.H. Mordhorst, N.C. Helm-Petersen, B.S. Hansen, J. Thârup, A. Poulsen, M. Sodemann, and M. Jakobsen
1989   Child mortality related to seroconversion or lack of seroconversion after measles vaccination. *Pediatric Infectious Disease Journal* 8(4):197-200.

Aaby, P., J. Bukh, D. Kronborg, I.M. Lisse, and M.C. da Silva
1990a   Delayed excess mortality after exposure to measles during the first six months of life. *American Journal of Epidemiology* 132(2):211-291.

Aaby, P., K. Knudsen, T.G. Jensen, J. Thârup, A. Poulsen, M. Sodemann, M.C. da Silva, and H. Whittle
1990b   Measles incidence, vaccine efficacy, and mortality in two urban African areas with high vaccination coverage. *Journal of Infectious Diseases* 162(5):1043-1048.

Aaby, P., M. Andersen, and K. Knudsen.
1993   Excess mortality after early exposure to measles. *International Journal of Epidemiology* 22(1):156-162.

Abrutyn, E., and J.A. Berlin
1991   Intrathecal therapy in tetanus: A meta-analysis. *Journal of the American Medical Association* 266(16):2262-2267.

Administrative Committee on Coordination—Subcommittee on Nutrition, United Nations
1987   *First Report on the World Nutrition Situation.* New York: United Nations.

Adu, F.D., O.A.O. Akinwolere, O. Tomori, and L.N. Uche
1992   Low seroconversion rates to measles vaccine among children in Nigeria. *Bulletin of the World Health Organization* 70(4):457-460.

Agounke, A., M. Assogba, and K. Anipah
1989   *Enquête Démographique et de Santé au Togo 1988.* Lomé, Togo: Unite de Recherche Démographique, Direction de la Statistique, Direction Générale de la Santé; Columbia, Md.: Institute for Resource Development/Macro Systems, Inc.

Alderman, M.H., H.T. Laverde, and A.T. d'Souza
1978   Reduction of young child malnutrition and mortality in rural Jamaica. *Journal of Tropical Pediatrics* 24:7-11.

Alihonou, M.E.
1970   Le tétanos néo-natal en zone tropicale. *L'Enfance en Milieu Tropical* 62-63:11-13.

Alonso, P.L., K. March, and B.M. Greenwood
1987   The accuracy of the clinical histories given by mothers of seriously ill African children. *Annals of Tropical Paediatrics* 7:187-189.

Alonso, P.L., S.W. Lindsay, J.R.M. Armstrong, M. Conteh, A.G. Hill, P.H. David, G. Fegan, A. de Francisco, A.J. Hall, F.C. Shenton, K. Cham, and B.M. Greenwood
1991   The effect of insecticide-treated bed nets on mortality of Gambian children. *Lancet* 1499-1502.

American Association for the Advancement of Science
1991   *Malaria and Development in Africa: A Cross-Sectoral Approach.* Washington, D.C.: American Association for the Advancement of Science.

Ascoli, W., et al.
1967   Nutrition and infection field study in Guatemalan villages, 1959-1964. *Archives of Environmental Health* 15:439-449.

Ashworth, A., and R.G. Feachem
1985a   Interventions for the control of diarrhoeal diseases among young children: Weaning education. *Bulletin of the World Health Organization* 63(6):1115-1127.

1985b   Interventions for the control of diarrhoeal diseases among young children: Prevention of low birth weight. *Bulletin of the World Health Organization* 63(1):165-184.

Babaniyi, O.A., and B.D. Parakoyi
1989   Mortality from neonatal tetanus in Ilorin: Results of a community-based survey. *Journal of Tropical Pediatrics* 35(3):137-138.

Baertl, J.M., E. Morales, G. Verastegui, and G.G. Graham
1970   Diet supplementation for entire communities: Growth and mortality of infants and children. *American Journal of Clinical Nutrition* 23:707-715.

Bairagi, R., M.K. Chowdhury, Y.J. Kim, and G.T.C. Curlin
1985   Alternative anthropometric indicators of mortality. *American Journal of Clinical Nutrition* 42:296-306.

Bang, A.T., R.A. Bang, O. Tale, P. Sontakke, J. Solanki, R. Wargantiwar, and P. Kelzarkar
1990   Reduction of pneumonia mortality and total childhood mortality by means of community-based intervention trial in Gadchiroli, India. *Lancet* 201-206.

Bantje, H.
1983   Seasonal variations in birthweight distribution in Ikwiriri Village, Tanzania. *Journal of Tropical Pediatrics* 29:50-54.

Barclay, A.J.G., A. Foster, and A. Sommer
1987   Vitamin A supplements and mortality related to measles: A randomised clinical trial. *British Medical Journal* 294:261-324.

Bassett, M.T., P. Taylor, J. Bvirakare, F. Chiteka, and E. Govere
1991   Clinical diagnosis of malaria: Can we improve? *Journal of Tropical Medicine and Hygiene* 94:65-69.

Beaton, G.H., and H. Ghassemi
1982   Supplementary feeding programs for young children in developing countries. *American Journal of Clinical Nutrition* 35(4, supplement):863-916.

Beaton, G.H., R. Martorell, K.A. L'Abbé, B. Edmonston, G. McCabe, A.C. Ross, and B. Harvey
1992   *Effectiveness of Vitamin A Supplementation in the Control of Young Child Morbidity and Mortality in Developing Countries.* Toronto: University of Toronto.

Becker, S., F. Diop, and J.N. Thornton
1993   Infant and child mortality in two counties of Liberia: Results of a survey in 1988 and trends since 1984. *International Journal of Epidemiology* (forthcoming).

Benenson, A.S.
1985   *Control of Communicable Diseases in Man.* Washington, D.C.: American Public Health Association.

Bergevin, Y., C. Dougherty, and M.S. Kramer
1983   Do infant formula samples shorten the duration of breastfeeding? *Lancet* 1148-1151.

Billewicz, W.Z., and I.A. McGregor
1982   The demography of two West African (Gambian) villages, 1951-1975. *Journal of Biosocial Sciences* 13:219-240.

Biritwum, R.B., S. Isomura, A. Assoku, and S. Torigoe
1986   Growth and diarrheal disease surveillance in a rural Ghanaian pre-school child population. *Transactions of the Royal Society of Tropical Medicine and Hygiene* 80:208-213.

Björkman, A., M. Willcox, N. Marbiah, and D. Payne
1991   Susceptibility of *Plasmodium falciparum* to different doses of quinine in vivo and to quinine and quinidine in vitro in relation to chloroquine in Liberia. *Bulletin of the World Health Organization* 69(4):459-465.

Black, F.L., L.L. Berman, J.M. Borgño, R.A. Capper, A.A. Carvalho, C. Collins, O. Glover, Z. Hijazi, D.L. Jacobson, Y.-L. Lee, M. Libel, A.C. Linhare, C.A. Mendizabal-Morris, E. Simones, E. Siqueira-Campos, J. Stevenson, and N. Vecchi
1986   Geographic variation in infant loss of maternal measles antibody and in prevalence of rubella antibody. *American Journal of Epidemiology* 124(3):442-452.

Blacker, J.G.C., J. Mukiza-Gapere, M. Kibet, P. Airey, and L. Werner
1987   Mortality differentials in Kenya. Paper presented to the International Union for the Scientific Study of Population seminar on mortality and society in sub-Saharan Africa, Yaoundé, October 19-23.

Blin, P., H.G. Delolme, J.D. Heyraud, Y. Charpak, and L. Sentilhes
1986   Evaluation of the protective effect of BCG vaccination by a case-control study in Yaoundé, Cameroon. *Tubercle* 67:283-288.

Bloom, B.R., and T. Godal
1983   Selective primary health care: Strategies for control of diseases in the developing world. *Review of Infectious Diseases* 5(6):765-780.

Boerma, J.T., A.E. Sommerfelt, S.O. Rutstein, and G. Rojas
1990   *Immunization: Levels, Trends and Differentials.* Demographic and Health Surveys Comparative Studies, No. 1. Columbia, Md.: Institute for Resource Development/Macro Systems, Inc.

Boerma, J.T., A.E. Sommerfelt, and S.O. Rutstein
1991   *Childhood Morbidity and Treatment Patterns.* Demographic and Health Surveys Comparative Studies, No. 4. Columbia, Md.: Institute for Resource Development/ Macro International, Inc.

Böttinger, M., S. Litnivov, F. Assaad, H. Lundbeck, L. Heller, and E.G. Beausoleil
1981   Antibodies against poliomyelitis and measles viruses in immunized and unimmunized children, Ghana 1976-78. *Bulletin of the World Health Organization* 59(5):729-736.

Bradley, A.K., S.B.J. MacFarlane, J.B. Moody, H.M. Gilles, J.G.C. Blacker, and B.D. Musa
1982   Malumfashi endemic diseases research project, XX; Demographic findings: Mortality. *Annals of Tropical Medicine and Parasitology* 76(4):393-404.

Bradley, D.J.
1991a   Morbidity and mortality at Pare-Taveta, Kenya and Tanzania, 1954-66: The effects of a period of malaria control. Pp. 248-263 in R.G. Feachem and D.T. Jamison, eds., *Disease and Mortality in Sub-Saharan Africa.* New York: Oxford University Press for The World Bank.
1991b   Malaria. Pp. 190-202 in R.G. Feachem and D.T. Jamison, eds., *Disease and Mortality in Sub-Saharan Africa.* New York: Oxford University Press for The World Bank.

Briend, A., M. Garenne, B. Maire, O. Fontaine, and K. Dieng
1989   Nutritional status, age and survival: The muscle mass hypothesis. *European Journal of Clinical Nutrition* 43:715-726.

Brinkman, U., and A. Brinkman
1991   Malaria and health in Africa: The present situation and epidemiological trends. *Tropical Medicine and Parasitology* 42(3):204-213.

Broome, C.V., S.R. Preblud, B. Bruner, J.E. McGowan, P.S. Hayes, B.P. Harris, W. Elssea, and D.W. Fraser
1981   Epidemiology of pertussis. Atlanta, 1977. *Journal of Pediatrics* 98:362-367.

Brown, J.E., and R.C. Brown
1979   An evaluation of nutrition centre effectiveness by measurement of younger siblings. *Transactions of the Royal Society of Tropical Medicine and Hygiene* 73:70-73.

Brown, K.H., A. Gaffar, and S.M. Alamgir
1979   Xerophthalmia, protein-calorie malnutrition, and infections in children. *Journal of Paediatrics* 95:651-656.

Burgess, W., B. Mduma, and G.V. Josephson
1986   Measles in Mbeya, Tanzania—1981-1983. *Journal of Tropical Pediatrics* 32:148-153.

Bwibo, N.O.
1971   The role of neonatal infection in neonatal and childhood mortality. *Journal of Tropical and Environmental Child Health* 17(3):89-90.
Campbell, C.C.
1991   Challenges facing antimalarial therapy in Africa. *Journal of Infectious Diseases* 163:1207-1211.
Cantrelle, P.
1968   Mortalité par rougeole dans la région du siné-saloum (Sénégal) 1963-1965. *L'Enfance en Milieu Tropical* 52:37-40.
1974   *La Méthode d'Observation Suivie par Enquète à Passages Répétés.* Chapel Hill, N.C.: Laboratories for Population Statistics, University of North Carolina.
Cantrelle, P.D., I.L. Diop, M. Garenne, M. Gueye, and A. Sadio
1986   The profile of mortality and its determinants in Senegal, 1960-1980. Pp. 86-116 in *Determinants of Mortality Change and Differentials in Developing Countries: The Five-Country Case Study Project.* United Nations Population Studies 94. New York: United Nations.
Carnell, M.A., and A.B. Guyon
1990   Nutritional status, migration, mortality, and measles vaccine coverage during the 1983-1985 drought period: Timbuktu, Mali. *Journal of Tropical Pediatrics* 36(3):109-113.
Centers for Disease Control
1983   Annual Summary, 1982. *Morbidity and Mortality Weekly Report* 31(supplement 1)(54):1-149.
1991   *Africa Child Survival Initiative: Combatting Childhood Communicable Diseases 1990-1991 Bilingual Annual Report.* Atlanta, Ga.: U.S. Government Printing Office.
Chahnazarian, A., D. Ewbank, B. Makani, and K. Ekouevi
1993   Impact of selective primary care on childhood mortality in a rural health zone of Zaire. *International Journal of Epidemiology* (forthcoming).
Chen, L.C., A. Chowdhury, and S.L. Huffman
1980   Anthropometric assessment of energy-protein malnutrition and subsequent risk of mortality among preschool aged children. *American Journal of Clinical Nutrition* 33:1836-1845.
Chen, L.C., M. Rahman, S. D'Souza, J. Chakraborty, A.M. Sardar, and M. Yunus
1983   Mortality impact of an MCH-FP program in Matlab, Bangladesh. *Studies in Family Planning* 14:199-209.
Cherry, J.D.
1984   The epidemiology of pertussis and pertussis immunization in the United Kingdom and the United States: A comparative study. *Current Problems in Pediatrics* 14(2):1-78.
Chieh-Johnson, D., A. Cross, A. Way, and J. Sullivan
1988   *Liberia Demographic and Health Survey 1986.* Monrovia, Liberia: Bureau of Statistics; Columbia, Md.: Institute for Resource Development/Westinghouse.
Chorlton, R.
1989   In F. Moneti, ed., *Improving Child Survival and Nutrition. The Joint WHO/UNICEF Nutrition Support Programme in Iringa, Tanzania.* Dar es Salaam, Tanzania: UNICEF.
Claeson, M., and M.H. Merson
1990   Global progress in the control of diarrheal diseases. *Pediatric Infectious Disease Journal* 9:345-355.

Clemens, J.D., B.F. Stanton, J. Chakraborty, and S. Chowdhury
1988   Measles vaccination and childhood mortality in rural Bangladesh. *American Journal of Epidemiology* 128(6):1330-1339.

Coale, A.J., and F. Lorimer
1967   Summary of estimates of fertility and mortality. In W. Brass and A.J. Coale, eds., *The Demography of Tropical Africa*. Princeton, N.J.: Princeton University Press.

Cohen, B.
1993   Fertility levels, differentials, and trends. In K. Foote, K. Hill, and L. Martin, eds., *Demographic Change in Sub-Saharan Africa*. Panel on the Population Dynamics of Sub-Saharan Africa, Committee on Population. Washington, D.C.: National Academy Press.

Cole-King, S.M.
1975   Under-fives clinic in Malawi. The development of a national programme. *Journal of Tropical Pediatrics* 21:183-191.

Cot, M., A. Roisin, D. Barro, A. Tada, J.-P. Verhave, P. Carnevale, and G. Breart
1992   Effect of chloroquine chemoprophylaxis during pregnancy on birth weight: Results of a randomized trial. *American Journal of Tropical Medicine and Hygiene* 46(1):21-27.

Coutsoudis, A., M. Broughton, and H. Coovadia
1991   Vitamin A supplementation reduces measles morbidity in young African children: A randomized, placebo-controlled double-blind trial. *American Journal of Clinical Nutrition* 54:890-895.

Cutts, F.T.
1988   The use of the WHO cluster survey method for evaluating the impact of the Expanded Programme on Immunization on target disease incidence. *Journal of Tropical Medicine and Hygiene* 91:231-239.

Cutts, F.T., P.G. Smith, S. Colombo, G. Mann, A. Ascherio, and A.C. Soares
1990a   Field evaluation of measles vaccine efficacy in Mozambique. *American Journal of Epidemiology* 131(2):349-355.

Cutts, F., A. Soares, A. Jecque, J. Cliff, S. Kortbeek, and S. Colombo
1990b   The use of evaluation to improve the Expanded Programme on Immunization in Mozambique. *Bulletin of the World Health Organization* 68(2):199-208.

Cutts, F.T., R.H. Henderson, C.J. Clements, R.T. Chen, and P.A. Patriarca
1991   Principles of measles control. *Bulletin of World Health Organization* 69(1):1-7.

Dabis, F., A. Sow, R.J. Waldman, P. Bikaiouri, J. Senga, G. Madzou, and T.S. Jones
1988   The epidemiology of measles in a partially vaccinated population in an African city: Implications for immunization programs. *American Journal of Epidemiology* 127(1):171-178.

Dan, V., A. Debroise, J.M. Zucker, and P. Satge
1971   Importance du tétanos néo-natal au Sénégal. *African Journal of Medical Science* 2:391-397.

Datta, N., V. Kumar, L. Kumar, and S. Singhi
1987   Application of case management to the control of acute respiratory infections in low-birth-weight infants: A feasibility study. *Bulletin of the World Health Organization* 65(1):77-82.

Daulaire, N.M.P., E.S. Starbuck, R.M. Houston, M.S. Church, T.A. Stukel, and M.R. Pandey
1992   Childhood mortality after a high dose of vitamin A in a high risk population. *British Medical Journal* 304:207-210.

De Graft-Johnson, K.T.
1988   Demographic data collection in Africa. In E. van de Walle, P.O. Ohadike, and

M.D. Sala-Diakanda, eds., *The State of African Demography*. Liège: International Union for the Scientific Study of Population.

Deming, M.S., A. Gayibor, K. Murphy, T.S. Jones, and T. Karsa
1989   Home treatment of febrile children with antimalarial drugs in Togo. *Bulletin of the World Health Organization* 67(6):695-700.

Deming, M.S., O.J. Kebba, M.W. Otten, E.W. Falgg, M. Jallow, M. Chan, D. Brogan, and H. N'jie
1992   Epidemic poliomyelitis in the Gambia following the control of poliomyelitis as an endemic disease. II. Clinical efficacy of trivalent oral polio vaccine. *American Journal of Epidemiology* 135(4):393-408.

De Sole, G., Y. Belay, and B. Zegeye
1987   Vitamin A deficiency in southern Ethiopia. *American Journal of Clinical Nutrition* 45:780-784.

de Swardt, R., C.B. Ijsselmuiden, and S. Johnson
1990   Vaccination status and seroprevalence of measles and polio antibodies in 1-6-year-old children in the Elim health ward of Gazankulu. *South African Medical Journal* 78(12):726-728.

De Vaquera, M.V., J.W. Townsend, J.J. Arroyo, and A. Lechtig
1983   The relationship between arm circumference at birth and early mortality. *Journal of Tropical Pediatrics* 29:167-174.

Draper, C.C.
1962   Studies in Malaria in Man in Africa. Unpublished thesis, University of Oxford, Oxford, United Kingdom.

Draper, C.C., J.L.M. Lelijveld, Y.G. Matola, and G.B. White
1972   Malaria in the Pare area of Tanzania. IV. Malaria in the human population 11 years after the suspension of residual insecticide spraying, with special reference to the serological findings. *Transaction of the Royal Society of Tropical Medicine and Hygiene* 66(6):905-912.

Einterz, E.M., and M.E. Bates
1991   Caring for neonatal tetanus patients in a rural primary care setting in Nigeria: A review of 237 cases. *Journal of Tropical Pediatrics* 37:179-181.

El-Rafie, M., W.A. Hassouna, N. Hirschhorn, and S. Loza
1990   Effect of diarrhoeal disease control on infant and childhood mortality in Egypt. *Lancet* (i):334-338.

El Samani, E.F.Z., W.C. Willett, and J.H. Ware
1988   Association of malnutrition and diarrhea in children aged under 5 years: A prospective follow-up study in a rural Sudanese community. *American Journal of Epidemiology* 128:93-105.

Embree, J.E., P. Datta, W. Stackiw, L. Sekla, M. Braddick, J.K. Kreiss, H. Pamba, I. Wamola, J.O. Ndinya-Achola, B.J. Law, P. Piot, K.K. Homes, and F.A. Plummer
1992   Increased risk of early measles in infants of human immunodeficiency virus type 1-seropositive mothers. *Journal of Infectious Diseases* 165(2):262-267.

European Collaborative Study
1991   Children born to women with HIV-1 infection: Natural history and risk of transmission. *Lancet* 253-260.

Ewbank, D.C., and S. Zimicki
1988   Implications of differences in the cause-structure of mortality for the design of health interventions. Paper presented at the conference on Child Survival Programs: Issues for the 1990s, Johns Hopkins School of Hygiene and Public Health, Baltimore, Md., November.

Ewbank, D.C., R. Henin, and J. Kekovole
1986   An integration of demographic and epidemiologic research on mortality in Kenya. Pp. 33-85 in *Determinants of Mortality Change and Differentials in Developing Countries*. New York: United Nations.
Expanded Programme on Immunization
1982   The opitmal age for measles immunization. *Weekly Epidemiological Record* 57(12):89-91.
1983   Neonatal tetanus mortality survey—Malawi. *Weekly Epidemiological Record* 58(42):326-327.
1986   Nosocomial measles. *Weekly Epidemiological Record* 61:338-340.
1989   Programme review—Malawi. *Weekly Epidemiological Record* 64(44):339-343.
1990   Rapid assessment of serological response to oral polio vaccine. *Weekly Epidemiological Record* 65(5):34-35.
1991   Measles outbreak, Kampala. *Weekly Epidemiological Record* 66(49):364-367.
1992   EPI Semiannual Update. WHO/EPI/CEIS/92.1. Geneva: World Health Organization
Farah, A-A., and S.H. Preston
1982   Child-mortality differentials in Sudan. *Population and Development Review* 8(2):365-383.
Fargues, P., and O. Nassour
1988   *Douze ans de Mortalité Urbaine au Sahel*. Travaux et Documents 123. Paris: Institut National d'Etudes Démographiques.
Fauveau, V., M. Yunus, K. Zaman, J. Chakraborty, and A.M. Sarder
1991   Diarrhoea mortality in rural Bangladeshi children. *Journal of Tropical Pediatrics* 37:31-36.
Fauveau, V., M.K. Stewart, J. Chakraborty, and S.A. Khan
1992   Mortality impact of a community-based programme to control acute lower respiratory tract infections. *Bulletin of the World Health Organization* 70(1):109-116.
Feachem, R.G.
1987   Vitamin A deficiency and diarrhoea: A review of interrelationships and their implications for the control of xerophthalmia and diarrhoea. *Tropical Diseases Bulletin* 84(3):R2-R15.
Feachem, R.G., and M.A. Koblinsky
1983   Interventions for the control of diarrhoeal disease among young children: Measles immunization. *Bulletin of the World Health Organization* 61(4):641-652.
1984   Interventions for the control of diarrhoeal diseases among young children: Promotion of breast-feeding. *Bulletin of the World Health Organization* 62(2):271-291.
Feery, B.J.
1984   Pertussis vaccine controversy: To vaccinate or not? *Austrian Pediatrics Journal* 20:91-93.
Fine, P.E.M.
1988   BCG vaccination against tuberculosis and leprosy. *British Medical Bulletin* 44(3):691-703.
Fine, P.E.M., and J.A. Clarkson
1984   Distribution of immunity to pertussis in the population of England and Wales. *Journal of Hygiene (Cambridge)* 92:21-26.
Fine, P.E.M., and J.M. Pönnighaus
1988   Leprosy in Malawi: 2. Background, design and prospects of the Karonga Prevention Trial, a leprosy vaccine trial in northern Malawi. *Transactions of the Royal Society Tropical Medicine and Hygiene* 82:810-817.

Fine, P.E.M., J.M. Pönnighaus, N. Maine, J.A. Clarkson, and L. Bliss
  1986   Protective efficacy of BCG against leprosy in northern Malawi. *Lancet* 499-502.
Fischer, P.R.
  1988   Measles in Zaire: 1987. *Clinical Pediatrics* 27(5):234-235.
Fleming, A.F., G.B.S. Ghatoura, K.A. Harrison, N.D. Briggs, and D.T. Dunn
  1986   The prevention of anaemia in pregnancy in primigravidae in the Guinea savanna of
          Nigeria. *Annals of Tropical Medicine and Parasitology* 80(2):211-233.
Foege, W.
  1971   Measles vaccination in Africa. Pp. 207-212 in *Proceedings of the International
          Conference on the Application of Vaccines against Viral, Rickettsial, and Bacte-
          rial Disease in Man.* Pan American Health Organization Scientific Publication
          226. Washington, D.C.: Pan American Health Organization.
Foster, S.O.
  1985   Ten priorities for child health. Pp. 97-110 in D.B. Jelliffe and E.F.P. Jelliffe, eds.,
          Advances in International Maternal and Child Health. New York: Oxford Uni-
          versity Press for The World Bank.
Foster, S.O., R.A. Spiegel, A. Mokdad, S. Yeanon, S.R. Becker, J. Thornton, and M.K. Galakpai
  1993   Immunization, oral rehydration therapy, and malaria chemotherapy, under-five children
          in Bomi and Grand Cape Mount Counties, Liberia, 1984 and 1988. *International
          Journal of Epidemiology* (forthcoming).
Freese, J.A., M.B. Markus, and J. Golenser
  1991   In vitro sensitivity of southern African reference isolates of *Plasmodium falciparum*
          to chloroquine and pyrimethamine. *Bulletin of the World Health Organization*
          69(6):707-712.
Gardiner, C., R.J. Biggar, W.E. Collins, and F.K. Nkrumah
  1984   Malaria in urban and rural areas of southern Ghana: A survey of parasitaemia,
          antibodies, and antimalarial practices. *Bulletin of the World Health Organization*
          62(4):607-613.
Gareaballah, E.-T., and B.P. Loevinsohn
  1989   The accuracy of mothers' reports about their children's vaccination status. *Bulletin
          of the World Health Organization* 67(6):669-674.
Garenne, M.
  1981   *The Age Pattern of Infant and Child Mortality in Rural West Africa.* Philadelphia:
          Population Studies Center, University of Pennsylvania.
Garenne, M., and P. Aaby
  1990   Pattern of exposure and measles mortality in Senegal. *Journal of Infectious Dis-
          eases* 161:1088-1094.
Garenne, M., and P. Cantrelle
  1986   Rougeole et mortalité au Sénégal: Etude de l'impact de la vaccination éffectué à
          Khombole 1965-1968 sur la survie des enfants. Pp. 515-532 in *Estimation de la
          Mortalité du Jeune Enfant (0-5 ans) pour Guider les Actions de Santé dans les
          Pays en Développement.* Séminarie méthodologique. CIE-INSERM-ORSTOM-
          INED, 145. Paris: INSERM.
Garenne, M., and O. Fontaine
  1986   Assessing probable cause of death using a standardized questionnaire: A study in
          rural Senegal. International Union for the Scientific Study of Population seminar
          on morbidity and mortality, Siena.
  1990   Assessing probable causes of death using a standardized questionnaire: A study in
          rural Senegal. In J. Vallin, S. D'Souza, and A. Palloni, eds., *Measurement and
          Analysis of Mortality: New Approaches.* Oxford: Clarendon Press.

Garenne, M., P. Cantrelle, and I. Diop
  1985   The case of Senegal. Pp. 315-340 in J. Vallin and A.D. Lopez, eds., *Health Policy, Social Policy and Mortality Prospects.* Liège: Ordina.
Garenne, M., L. Odile, J.P. Beau, and I. Sene
  1991   Child mortality after high-titre measles vaccines in Senegal: Response. *Lancet* 1518-1519.
Garenne, M., O. Leroy, J.-P. Beau, and I. Sene
  1992   *Clinical Efficacy of Measles Vaccines in Niakhar, a Rural Area of Senegal.* Department of Population and International Health, Harvard School of Public Health, Boston, Mass.
Gascon, J., A. Merlos, N. Madrenys, J.M. Torres, and J.L. Bada
  1988   Epidemiology of malaria in Nyarutova (Rwanda): A clinical, parasitological and serological study. *Transactions of the Royal Society of Tropical Medicine and Hygiene* 82(2):222.
Ghana Health Assessment Team
  1981   A quantitative method of assessing the health impact of different diseases in less developed countries. *International Journal of Epidemiology* 10(1):73-80.
Ghana Statistical Service and Institute for Resource Development
  1989   *Ghana Demographic and Health Survey 1988.* Accra, Ghana: Ghana Statistical Services; Columbia, Md.: Institute for Resource Development/Macro Systems, Inc.
Gilles, H.M., J.B. Lawson, M. Sibelas, A. Voller, and N. Allan
  1969   Malaria, anaemia and pregnancy. *Annals of Tropical Medicine and Parasitology* 63(2):245-262.
Glass, R., and R.E. Black
  1992   Epidemiology of cholera. Pp. 129-154 in D. Barua and W.B. Greenough, III, eds., *Cholera.* New York: Plenum Medical Book Co.
Goh-Rowland, S.G.J., N. Lloyd-Evans, K. Williams, and M.G.M. Rowland
  1985   The etiology of diarrhoea studied in the community in young urban Gambian children. *Journal of Diarrhoeal Disease Research* 3:7-13.
Gomez, F., R. Galvan, S. Frenk, J.C. Munoz, R. Chavez, and J. Vasquez
  1956   Mortality in second and third degree malnutrition. *Journal of Tropical Pediatrics* 2:77.
Gracey, M., G. Cullity, and S. Suharjono
  1977   The stomach in malnutrition. *Archives of Disease in Childhood* 52:325-327.
Gray, R., G. Smith, and P. Barss
  1990   *The Use of Verbal Autopsy Methods to Determine Selected Causes of Death in Children.* Occasional Paper No. 10. Baltimore, Md.: Institute for International Programs, Johns Hopkins University.
Greenwood, B.M., and H. Pickering
  1993   A malaria control trial using insecticide-treated bednets and targeted chemoprophylaxis in a rural area of The Gambia, West Africa. 1. A review of the epidemiology and control of malaria in The Gambia. *Transactions of the Royal Society of Tropical Medicine and Hygiene* 87 (special supplement) forthcoming.
Greenberg, A.E., M. Ntumbanzondo, N. Ntula, L. Mawa, J. Howell, and F. Davachi
  1989   Hospital-based surveillance of malaria-related paediatric morbidity and mortality in Kinshasa, Zaire. *Bulletin of the World Health Organization* 67:189-196.
Greenwood, B.M., A.K. Bradley, A.M. Greenwood, P. Byass, K. Jammeh, K. Marsh, S. Tullock, F.S.J. Oldfield, and R. Hayes
  1987   Mortality and morbidity from malaria among children in a rural area of the Gambia,

West Africa. *Transactions of the Royal Society of Tropical Medicine and Hygiene* 81:478-486.

Greenwood, B.M., A.M. Greenwood, A.K. Bradley, R.W. Snow, P. Byass, R.J. Hayes, and A.B. Hatib-N'Jie
1988   Comparison of two strategies for control of malaria within a primary health care programme in the Gambia. *Lancet* (i):1121-1126.

Greenwood, B.M., A.M. Greenwood, R.W. Snow, P. Byass, S. Bennett, and A.B. Hatib-N'Jie
1989   The effects of malaria chemoprophylaxis given by traditional birth attendants on the course and outcome of pregnancy. *Transactions of the Royal Society of Tropical Medicine and Hygiene* 83:589-594.

Greenwood, B.M., A.K. Bradley, P. Byass, A.M. Greenwood, A. Menon, R.W. Snow, R.J. Hayes, and A.B. Hatib-N'Jie
1990   Evaluation of a primary health care programme in the Gambia. II. Its impact on mortality and morbidity in young children. *Journal of Tropical Medicine and Hygiene* 93:87-97.

Habicht, J.-P., and P.A. Berman
1980   Planning primary health services from a body count? *Social Science and Medicine* 14C:129-136.

Hamill, P.V.V., T.A. Drizd, C.L. Johnson, R.B. Reed, and A.F. Roche
1977   *NCHS Growth Curves for Children, Birth-18 Years, United States.* DHEW Pub. No. (PHS) 78-1650. Hyattsville, Md.: National Center for Health Statistics.

Hamilton, P.J.S., D.A.M. Gebbie, N.E. Wilks, and F. Lothe
1972   The role of malaria, folic acid deficiency and haemoglobin AS in pregnancy at Mulago hospital. *Transactions of the Royal Society of Tropical Medicine and Hygiene* 66(4):594-602.

Hanlon, P., B. Byass, M. Yamuah, R. Hayes, S. Bennett, and B.H. M'Boge
1988   Factors influencing vaccination compliance in peri-urban Gambian children. *Journal of Tropical Medicine and Hygiene* 91:29-33.

Heligman, L., N. Chen, and O. Babokol
1993   Shifts in the structure of population and deaths in less developed regions. In J. Gribble and S. Preston, ed., *The Epidemiological Transition: Policy and Planning Implications.* Washington, D.C.: National Academy Press.

Herrera, M.G., P. Nestel, A. El Amin, W.W. Fawzi, K.A. Mohamed, and L. Weld
1992   Vitamin A supplementation and child survival. *Lancet* 267-271.

Heymann, D.L., G.K. Mayben, K.R. Murphy, B.F. Stanley, and O. Guyer
1983   Measles control in Yaoundé: Justification of a one dose, nine months minimum age vaccination policy in tropical Africa. *Lancet* (i):1470-1472.

Heymann, D.L., R.W. Steketee, J.J. Wirima, D.A. McFarland, C.O. Khoromana, and C.C. Campbell
1990   Antenatal chloroquine chemoprophylaxis in Malawi: Chloroquine resistance, compliance, protective efficacy and cost. *Transactions of the Royal Society of Tropical Medicine and Hygiene* 84(4):496-498.

Hill, A.L.L.
1991   Infant and child mortality: Levels, trends and data deficiencies. In R. Feachem and D. Jamison, eds., *Disease and Mortality in Sub-Saharan Africa.* New York: Oxford University Press for The World Bank.
1992   Trends in childhood mortality in sub-Saharan mainland Africa. In G. Pison, E. van de Walle, and M. Sala-Diakanda, eds., *Mortality and Society in Sub-Saharan Africa.* Oxford: Clarendon Press.

Hill, A.L.L., and K. Hill
1988   Mortality in Africa: Levels, trends, differentials and prospects. In E. van de

Walle, P. O. Ohadike, and D. Sala-Diakanda, eds., *The State of African Demography*. Liège: International Union for the Scientific Study of Population.

Hinman, A.R.
1984   The pertussis vaccine controversy. *Public Health Reports* 99:255-259.

Hinman, A.R., and J.P. Koplan
1984   Pertussis and pertussis vaccine. Reanalysis of benefits, risks, and costs. *Journal of the American Medical Association* 251(23):3109-3113.

Hinman, A., S. Wassilah, and K. Bart
1986   Pertussis. In J.M. Last, ed., *Public Health and Preventive Medicine*. Norwalk, Conn.: Appleton-Century-Crofts.

Hobcraft, J., J. MacDonald, and S. Rutstein
1985   Demographic determinants of infant and early child mortality: A comparative analysis. *Population Studies* 38:363-385.

Hoorveg, J., and I. McDowell
1979   *Evaluation of Nutrition Education in Africa*. The Hague: Mouton.

Huffman, S.L., B.A.C. Yeager, R.E. Levine, J. Shelton, and M. Labbok
1991   *Breastfeeding Saves Lives: An Estimate of the Impact of Breastfeeding on Infant Mortality in Developing Countries*. Bethesda, Md.: NURTURE/Center to Prevent Childhood Malnutrition.

Hull, H.F.
1988   Increased measles mortality in households with multiple cases in the Gambia, 1981. *Review of Infectious Diseases* 10(2):453-457.

Hull, H.F., P.J. Williams, and F. Oldfield
1983   Measles mortality and vaccine efficacy in rural West Africa. *Lancet* (i):972-1075.

Hussey, G.D., and M. Klein
1990   A randomized, controlled trial of vitamin A in children with severe measles. *New England Journal of Medicine* 323(3):160-164.

International Science and Technology Institute
1990   Standard Report, November 1990. Center for International Health Information, Arlington, Va.

Irgens, L.M., and R. Skjaerven
1985   Secular trends in age at onset, sex ratio, and type index in leprosy observed during declining incidence rates. *American Journal of Epidemiology* 122:695-705.

Jelliffe, D.
1966   *The Assessment of the Nutritional Status of the Community*. Geneva: World Health Organization.

Kaijuka, E.M., E Kaija, A. Cross, and E. Loaiza
1989   *Uganda Demographic and Health Survey 1988/1989*. Entebbe, Uganda: Ministry of Health; Columbia, Md.: Institute for Resource Development.

Kalter, H.D., R.H. Gray, R.E. Black, and A. Gultiano
1990   Validation of post-mortem interviews to ascertain selected causes of death in children. *International Journal of Epidemiology* 19:380-386.

Kambarami, R.A., K.J. Nathoo, F.K. Nkrumah, and D.J. Pirie
1991   Measles epidemic in Harare, Zimbabwe, despite high measles immunization coverage rates. *Bulletin of the World Health Organization* 69(2):213-219.

Kandeh, B.S.
1986   Causes of infant and early childhood deaths in Sierra Leone. *Social Science and Medicine* 23(3):297-303.

Kaseje, D.C., and E.K.N. Sempebwa
1989   An integrated rural health project in Saradidi, Kenya. *Social Science and Medicine* 28(10):1063-1071.

Kasongo Project Team
1981   Influence of measles vaccination on survival pattern of 7-35-month-old children in Kasongo, Zaire. *Lancet* 764-767.
1983   Anthropometric assessment of young children's nutritional status as an indicator of subsequent risk of dying. *Journal of Tropical Pediatrics* 29:69-75.
1986   Growth decelerations among under-5-year-old children in Kasongo (Zaire). I. Occurrence of decelerations and impact of measles on growth. *Bulletin of the World Health Organization* 64(5):695-701.

Katende, C.
1992   The effect of accessibility to clinic on infant mortality in Africa: The cases of Liberia and Zimbabwe. Commissioned paper for the Working Group on the Effects of Child Survival and General Health Programs on Mortality, Panel on the Population Dynamics of Sub-Saharan Africa, Committee on Population, National Research Council, Washington, D.C.

Kennedy, E.
1991   *Successful Nutrition Programs in Africa: What Makes Them Work?* Policy, Research, and External Affairs Working Papers. Washington, D.C.: The World Bank.

Kenya Bureau of Statistics
1979   *Child Nutrition in Kenya.* Nairobi: UNICEF.

Kenya Ministry of Health
1978   Health information system in-patient report, 1978. *Health Information Bulletin (Nairobi)* 4(4):3-18.
1982   *A Report by the Director of Medical Services on Status of Health in Kenya, 1979.* Nairobi: Government Printing Office.

Kenya Ministry of Health and World Health Organization
1977   Measles immunity in the first year after birth and the optimum age for vaccination in Kenyan children. *Bulletin of the World Health Organization* 55:21-31.

Kenyan National Council for Population and Development and Institute for Resource Development
1989   *Kenya Demographic and Health Survey 1989.* Nairobi, Kenya: National Council for Population and Development; Columbia, Md.: Institute for Resource Development/Macro Systems, Inc.

Khan, A.J., J.A. Khan, M. Akbar, and D.G. Addiss
1990   Acute respiratory infections in children: A case management intervention in Abbottabad District, Pakistan. *Bulletin of the World Health Organization* 68(5):577-585.

Kielmann, A.A., and C. McCord
1978   Weight-for-age as an index of risk of death in children. *Lancet* 1247-1250.

Kielmann, A.A., A.B. Mobarek, M.T. Hammany, A.I. Gomma, A. El-Saad, R.K. Lotfi, I. Mazen, and A. Nagaty
1985   Control of deaths from diarrheal disease in rural communities. I. Design of an intervention study and effects on child mortality. *Tropical Medicine and Parasitology* 36:191-198.

Killewo, J., C. Makwaya, E. Munubhi, and R. Mpembeni
1991   The protective effect of measles vaccine under routine vaccination conditions in Dar es Salaam, Tanzania: A case-control study. *International Journal of Epidemiology* 20(2):508-514.

Kimati, V.P., and B. Lyaruu
1976   Measles complications as seen at Mwanza Regional Consultant and Teaching Hospital in 1973. *East African Medical Journal* 53(6):332-340.

Kirkwood, B.R.
1991   Acute respiratory infections. Pp. 158-172 in R.G. Feachem and D.T. Jamison,

eds., *Disease and Mortality in Sub-Saharan Africa*. New York: Oxford University Press for The World Bank.

Klaus, N.H., and J.H. Kennell
1976   *Maternal-Infant Bonding*. St. Louis, Mo.: The C.V. Mosby Co.

Koenig, M.A.
1992   Mortality reductions from measles and tetanus immunizations: A review of the evidence. Pp. 43-72 in K. Hill, ed., *Child Health Priorities for the 1990s*. Baltimore, Md.: The Johns Hopkins University Institute for International Program.

Koenig, M.A., M.A. Khan, B. Wojtyniak, J.D. Clemens, J. Chakraborty, V. Fauveau, J.F. Phillips, J. Akbar, and U.S. Barua
1990   Impact of measles vaccination on childhood mortality in rural Bangladesh. *Bulletin of the World Health Organization* 68(4):441-448.

Kofoed, P.E.L., and G. Simonsen
1988   Neonatal tetanus in Machakos, Kenya. *East African Medical Journal* 65(1):16-17.

Koster, F.T.
1988   Mortality among primary and secondary cases of measles in Bangladesh. *Review of Infectious Disease* 10(2):471-473.

Koster, F.T., G.C. Curlin, K.M. Aziz, and A. Haque
1981   Synergistic impact of measles and diarrhea on nutrition and mortality in Bangladesh. *Bulletin of the World Health Organization* 59:901-908.

Kramer, M.S.
1987   Determinants of low birthweight: Methodological assessment and meta-analysis. *Bulletin of the World Health Organization* 65:663-737.

Kumar, V., R. Kumar, and N. Datta
1987   Oral rehydration therapy in reducing diarrhoea-related mortality in rural India. *Journal of Diarrhoeal Disease Research* 5:159-164.

Kuming, B.S., and W.M. Politzer
1967   Xerophthalmia and protein malnutrition in Bantu children. *British Journal of Ophthalmology* 51:649-665.

Lamb, W.H.
1988   Epidemic measles in a highly immunized rural West African (Gambian) village. *Review of Infectious Diseases* 10(2):457-462.

Lamb, W.H., F.A. Foord, C.M.B. Lamb, and R.G. Whitehead
1984   Changes in maternal and child mortality rates in three isolated Gambian villages over ten years. *Lancet* 912-913.

Lancet
1984   Herd immunity to pertusis. Letter to the editor. *Lancet* (i):226-227.

Lang, T., C. Lafaix, D. Fassin, I. Arnaut, B. Salmon, D. Baudon, and J. Ezekiel
1986   Acute respiratory infections: A study of 151 children in Burkina Faso. *International Journal of Epidemiology* 15:553-561.

Lechtig, A., H. Delgado, C. Yarbrough, J.-P. Habicht, R. Martorell, and R.E. Klein
1975a   A simple assessment of the risk of low birthweight to select women for nutritional intervention. *American Journal of Obstetrics and Gynecology* 125:25-34.

Lechtig, A., J.-P. Habicht, H. Delgado, R.E. Klein, C. Yarbrough, and R. Martorell
1975b   Effect of food supplementation during pregnancy on birth weight. *Pediatrics* 56:508-520.

Leeuwenberg, J., W. Gembert, A.S. Muller, and S.C. Patel
1978   The incidence of diarrhoeal disease in the under-five population. *Tropical and Geographic Medicine* 30:383-391.

Leeuwenberg, J., A.S. Muller, A.M. Voorhoeve, W. Gemert, and P.W. Kok
1984   The epidemiology of measles. Pp. 77-94 in J.K. Van Ginneken and A.S. Muller,

eds., *Maternal and Child Health in Rural Kenya. An Epidemiological Study.* London: Croom Helm.

Leroy, O., and M. Garenne
1991   Risk factors of neonatal tetanus in Senegal. *International Journal of Epidemiology* 20(2):521-526.

Lindskog, U., P. Lindskog, J. Carstensen, and Y. Larsson
1988   Childhood mortality in relation to nutritional status and water supply—A prospective study from rural Malawi. *Acta Paediatrica Scandinavica* 77:260-268.

Lindtjorn, B.
1990   Famine in southern Ethiopia 1985-6: Population structure, nutritional state, and incidence of death among children. *British Medical Journal* 301:1123-1126.

Loevinsohn, B.P.
1990   The changing age structure of diphtheria patients: Evidence for the effectiveness of the EPI in the Sudan. *Bulletin of the World Health Organization* 68(3):353-357.

Markowitz, L.E., N. Nzilambi, W.J. Driskell, M.G. Sension, E.Z. Rovira, P. Nieburg, and R.W. Ryder
1989   Vitamin A levels and mortality among hospitalized measles patients, Kinshasa, Zaire. *Journal of Tropical Pediatrics* 35:109-112.

Maru, M., A. Getahun, and S. Hasana
1988   A house-to-house survey of neonatal tetanus in urban and rural areas in the Gondar Region, Ethiopia. *Tropical and Geographical Medicine* 40:233-236.

Mata, L.J.
1978   *The Children of Santa Maria Cauqué: A Prospective Field Study of Health and Growth.* Cambridge, Mass.: MIT Press.
1983   Promotion of breastfeeding, health, and growth among hospital-born neonates, and among infants of a rural area of Costa Rica. In L.C. Chen and N.S. Scrimshaw, eds., *Diarrhea and Malnutrition.* New York: Plenum Press.

Mbacké, C., and E. van de Walle
1992   Socio-economic factors and use of health services as determinants of child mortality. Pp. 123-144 in E. van de Walle, G. Pison, M. Sala-Diakanda, eds., *Mortality and Society in Sub-Saharan Africa.* Oxford: Clarendon Press.

Mbithi, P.M., and B. Wisner
1972   Drought and famine in Kenya: Magnitude and attempted solutions. Institute for Development Studies Discussion Paper No. 144, Nairobi.

Mburu, F.M., H.C. Spencer, and D.C.O. Kaseje
1987   Changes in sources of treatment occurring after inception of a community-based malaria control programme in Saradidi, Kenya. *Annals of Tropical Medicine and Parasitology* 81(supplement 1):105-110.

McDermott, J.M., D.L. Heymann, J.J. Wirima, A.P. Macheso, R.D. Wahl, R.W. Steketee, and C.C. Campbell
1988   Efficacy of chemoprophylaxis in preventing *Plasmodium falciparum* parasitaemia and placental infection in pregnant women in Malawi. *Transactions of the Royal Society of Tropical Medicine and Hygiene* 82:520-523.

McGregor, I.A.
1984   Epidemiology, malaria and pregnancy. *American Journal of Tropical Medicine and Hygiene* 33(4):517-525.
1991   Morbidity and mortality at Keneba, the Gambia, 1950-1975. Pp. 306-324 in R.G. Feachem and D.T. Jamison, eds., *Disease and Mortality in Sub-Saharan Africa.* New York: Oxford University Press for The World Bank.

Melgaard, B., G. Kimani, and D.M. Mutie
1987   A community study of neonatal tetanus in Kenya. *East African Medical Journal* 64(7):458-463.

Melgaard, B., D.M. Mutie, and G. Kimani
1988   A cluster survey of mortality due to neonatal tetanus in Kenya. *International Journal of Epidemiology* 17(1):174-177.

Menon, A., D. Joof, K.M. Rowan, and B.M. Greenwood
1988   Maternal administration of chloroquine: An unexplored aspect of malaria control. *Journal of Tropical Medicine and Hygiene* 91:49-54.

Menon, A., R.W. Snow, P. Byass, B.M. Greenwood, R.J. Hayes, and A.B. Hatib-N'Jie
1990   Sustained protection against mortality and morbidity from malaria in rural Gambian children by chemoprophylaxis given by village health workers. *Transactions of the Royal Society of Tropical Medicine and Hygiene* 84(6):768-772.

Merhai, Z., and A. Kumar
1986   Tetanus in infancy and childhood (a review of 110 cases from Addis Ababa, Ethiopia). *East African Medical Journal* 63(11):736-741.

Migliori, G.B., A. Borghesi, P. Rossanigo, C. Adriko, M. Neri, S. Santini, A. Bartoloni, F. Paradisi, and G. Acocella
1992   Proposal of an improved score method for diagnosis of pulmonary tuberculosis in childhood in developing countries. *Tubercle and Lung Disease* 73:145-149.

Miller, C.
1987   Live measles vaccine: A 21 year follow-up. *British Medical Journal* 295:22-24.

Miller, D.L., R. Alderslade, and E.M. Ross
1982   Whooping cough and whopping cough vaccine: The risks and benefits debate. *Epidemiologic Review* 4:1-24.

Miller, J.K.
1972   The prevention of neonatal tetanus by maternal immunization. *Journal of Tropical Pediatrics and Environmental Child Health* 18(2):159-167.

Molineaux, L.
1985   The impact of parasitic diseases and their control, with an emphasis on malaria and Africa. Pp. 13-44 in J. Vallin and A.D. Lopez, eds., *Health Policy, Social Policy and Mortality Prospects.* Liège: Ordina.

Molineaux, L., and G. Gramiccia
1980   *The Garki Project: Research on the Epidemiology and Control of Malaria in the Sudan Savanna of West Africa.* Geneva: World Health Organization.

Mongi, P.S., R.L. Mbise, A.E. Msengi, and D.M. Do Amsi
1987   Tetanus neonatorum—Experience with intrathecal serotherapy at Muhimbili Medical Centre, Dar es Salaam, Tanzania. *Annals of Tropical Paediatrics* 7(1):27-31.

Moran, J., and J. Bernard
1989   The spread of chloroquine-resistant malaria in Africa: Implications for travelers. *Journal of the American Medical Association* 262:245-258.

Morley, D.
1966   Whooping cough in Nigerian children. *Tropical and Geographical Medicine* 18:169-182.

Morley, D., M. Woodland, and W.F.J. Cuthbertson
1964   Controlled trial of pyrimethamine in pregnant women in an African village. *British Medical Journal* 1:667-668.

Mortimer, E.A.
1988   Pertussis vaccine. Pp. 74-97 in S.A. Plotkink and E.A. Mortimer, eds., *Vaccines.* Philadelphia: Saunders.

Mosley, W.H.
1988   Is there a middle way? Categorical programs for PHC. *Social Science and Medicine* 26(9):907-908.
Mtango, F.D.E., and D. Neuvians
1986   Acute respiratory infections in children under five years. Control project in Bagamoyo District, Tanzania. *Transactions of the Royal Society of Tropical Medicine and Hygiene* 80:851-858.
Muller, A.S., and J. Leeuwenburg
1985   *Epidemiology and Control of Whooping Cough.* Geneva: World Health Organization.
Muller, A.S., and J.K. van Ginneken
1991   Morbidity and mortality in Machakos, Kenya, 1974-81. Pp. 264-285 in R.G. Feachem and D.T. Jamison, eds., *Disease and Mortality in Sub-Saharan Africa.* New York: Oxford University Press for The World Bank.
Muller, A.S., A.M. Voorhoeve, W. t'Mannetje, and T.W.J. Schulpen
1977   The impact of measles in a rural area of Kenya. *East African Medical Journal* 54(7):364-373.
Muller, A.S., J. Leeuwenberg, and A.M. Voorhoeve
1984a   Pertussis in a rural area of Kenya: Epidemiology and results of a vaccine trial. *Bulletin of the World Health Organization* 62(6):899-908.
Muller, A.S., J. Leeuwenburg, and A.M. Voorhoeve
1984b   The epidemiology of pertussis and results of a vaccine trial. In J. van Ginneken and A.S. Muller, eds., *Maternal and Child Health in Rural Kenya.* London: Croom Helm.
Murray, C.J.L.
1991   Epidemiological and demographic evidence on the levels and trends in tuberculosis. Paper presented at the International Union for the Scientific Study of Population seminar on causes and prevention of adult mortality in developing countries, Santiago, October 7-11.
Murray, C.J.L., E. DeJonghe, H.J. Chum, D.S. Nyangulu, A. Salomao, and K. Styblo
1991   Cost effectiveness of chemotherapy for pulmonary tuberculosis in three sub-Saharan African countries. *Lancet* (ii):1305-1308.
Mutabingwa, T.K., L.N. Malle, and S.N. Mtui
1991   Chloroquine therapy still useful in the management of malaria during pregnancy in Muheza, Tanzania. *Tropical and Geographical Medicine* 43(1-2):131-135.
National Control of Diarrheal Diseases Project
1988   Impact of the national control of diarrhoeal diseases project on infant and child mortality in Dakahlia, Egypt. *Lancet*(ii):145-148.
Ndiaye, S., I. Sarr, and M. Ayad
1988   *Enquôte Démographique et de Santé au Senegal 1986.* Dakar, Sénégal: Ministère de l'Economie et de Finances; Columbia, Md.: Institute for Resource Development/Westinghouse.
Neumann, A.K., F.T. Sai, and S. Ofusu-Amaah
1991   The Danfa comprehensive rural health project, Ghana, 1969-79. Pp. 324-357 in R.G. Feachem and D.T. Jamison, eds., *Disease and Mortality in Sub-Saharan Africa.* New York: Oxford University Press for The World Bank.
Newell, K.W.
1988   Selective primary health care: The counter revolution. *Social Science and Medicine* 26(9):903-906.
Nigerian Federal Office of Statistics and Institute for Resource Development
1992   *Nigeria Demographic and Health Survey 1990.* Lagos, Nigeria: Federal Office of

Statistics; Columbia, Md.: Institute for Resource Development/Macro International, Inc.

Nougtara, A., R. Sauerborn, C. Oepen, and H.J. Diesfeld
1989 Assessment of MCH services offered by professional and community health workers in the district of Solenzo, Burkina Faso. I. Utilization of MCH services. *Journal of Tropical Pediatrics* 35(supplement 1):2-9.

Oakes, S., V. Mitchell, G. Pearson, and C. Carpenter, eds.
1991 *Malaria: Obstacles and Opportunities.* Committee for the Study on Malaria Prevention and Control: Status Review and Alternative Strategies, Division of International Health, Institue of Medicine. Washington, D.C.: National Academy Press.

Oberle, M.W., M.H. Merson, M.S. Islam, A.S.M. Rahman, D.H. Huber, and G. Curlin
1990 Diarrhoeal disease in Bangladesh: Epidemiology, mortality averted and costs at a rural treatment centre. *International Journal of Epidemiology* 9:341-348.

Oduntan, S.
1978 The immunological response of Nigerian infants to attenuated and inactivated polio-vaccines. *Annals of Tropical Medicine and Parasitology* 72:111-115.

Ofosu-Amaah, S.
1983 The control of measles in tropical Africa: A review of past and present efforts. *Reviews of Infectious Diseases* 5(3):546-553.

Ogbu, O., and M. Gallagher
1992 Public expenditures and health care in Africa. *Social Science and Medicine* 34(6):615-624.

Olivar, M., M. Develoux, A.C. Abari, and L. Loutan
1991 Presumptive diagnosis of malaria results in a significant risk of mistreatment of children in urban Sahel. *Transactions of the Royal Society of Tropical Medicine and Hygiene* 85(6)729-730.

Omondi-Odhiambo, J.K. van Ginneken, and A.M. Voorhoeve
1990 Mortality by cause of death in a rural area of Machakos District, Kenya in 1975-78. *Journal of Biosocial Sciences* 22(1):63-76.

Onyemunwa, P.
1988 Health care practices and use of health services as factors affecting child survival in Benin City, Nigeria. African Population Conference, Dakar, Senegal, November 7-12.

Orenstein, W.A., R.H. Bernier, T.J. Dondero, A.R. Hinman, J.S. Marks, K.J. Bart, and B. Sirotkin
1985 Field evaluation of vaccine efficacy. *Bulletin of the World Health Organization* 63(6):1055-1068.

Orenstein, W.A., A.R. Hinman, and K.J. Bart
1986 Measles. Pp. 157-161 in J.N. Last, ed., *Public Health and Preventive Medicine.* Norwalk, Conn.: Appleton-Century-Crofts.

Orofi-Adjei, D., J.O.O. Commey, and K.K. Adjepon-Yamoah
1984 Serum chloroquine levels in children before treatment for malaria (letter). *Lancet* i:1246.

Oruamabo, R.S., and C.T. John
1989 Antenatal care and fetal outcome, especially low birthweight, in Port Harcourt, Nigeria. *Annals of Tropical Paediatrics* 3:173-177.

Otten, M.W., M.S. Deming, K.O. Jaiteh, E.W. Flagg, I. Forgie, Y. Sanyang, B. Sillah, D. Brogan, and P. Gowers
1992 Epidemic poliomyelitis in the Gambia following the control of poliomyelitis as an endemic disease. I. Descriptive findings. *American Journal of Epidemiology* 135(4):381-392.

Owa, J.A., and O.O. Makinde
1990   Neonatal tetanus in babies of immunized mothers. *Journal of Tropical Pediatrics* 36:143-144.
Page, H.J., and A.J. Coale
1972   Fertility and child mortality south of the Sahara. Pp. 51-66 in S.H. Ominde and C.N. Ejiogu, eds., *Population Growth and Economic Development in Africa.* New York: Population Council.
Pandey, M.R., P.R. Sharma, B.B. Gubhaju, G.M. Shakya, R.P. Neupane, A. Gautam, and I.B. Shrestha
1989   Impact of a pilot acute respiratory infection (ARI) control programme in a rural community on the hill region of Nepal. *Annals of Tropical Paediatrics* 9:212-220.
Pandey, M.R., N.M.P. Daulaire, E.S. Starbuck, R.M. Houston, and K. McPherson
1991   Reduction in total under-five mortality in western Nepal through community-based antimicrobial treatment of pneumonia. *Lancet* 993-997.
Parker, R.L., W. Rinehart, P.T. Piotrow, and L. Doucette
1985   Oral rehydration therapy (ORT) for childhood diarrhea. *Population Reports: Issues in World Health* 12(4):41-75.
Patriarca, P.A., R.J. Biellik, G. Sanden, D.G. Burstyn, P.D. Mitchell, P.R. Silverman, J. P. Davis, and C.R. Manclark
1988   Sensitivity and specificity of clinical case definitions for pertussis. *American Journal of Public Health* 78(7):833-836.
Payne, D., B. Grab, R.E. Fontaine, and J.H.G. Hempel
1976   Impact of control measures on malaria transmission and general mortality. *Bulletin of the World Health Organization* 54:369-377.
Pelletier, D.L.
1991   *Relationships Between Child Anthropometry and Mortality in Developing Countries: Implications for Policy, Programs, and Future Research.* Ithaca, N.Y.: Cornell Food and Nutrition Policy Program.
Phillips, J.F., R. Simmons, J. Chakraborty, and A.I. Chowdhury
1984   Integrating health services into an MCH-FP program: Lessons from Matlab, Bangladesh. *Studies in Family Planning* 15:153-161.
Pison, G., and N. Bonneuil
1988   Increased risk of measles mortality for children with siblings among the Fula Bande, Senegal. *Review of Infectious Diseases* 10(2):468-470.
Pison, G., J.F. Trape, M. Lefebvre, and C. Enel
1993   Rapid decline in child mortality in a rural area of Senegal. *International Journal of Epidemiology* 22(1):72-80.
Pollock, T.M., E. Miller, and J. Lobb
1984   Severity of whooping cough in England before and after the decline in pertussis immunization. *Archives of Disease in Childhood* 59(2):162-165.
Pönnighaus, J.M., P.E.M. Fine, J.A.C. Sterne, R.J. Wilson, E. Msosa, P.J.K. Gruer, P.A. Jenkins, S.B. Lucas, N.G. Liomba, and L. Bliss
1992   Efficacy of BCG vaccine against leprosy and tuberculosis in northern Malawi. *Lancet* 339(i):636-639.
Porter, J.D., M. Gastellu-Etchegorry, I. Navarre, G. Lungu, and A. Moren
1990   Measles outbreaks in the Mozambican refugee camps in Malawi: The continued need for an effective vaccine. *International Journal of Epidemiology* 19(4):1072-1077.
Potter, J.E., O. Mojarro, and L. Nunuz
1987   The influence of maternal health care on the prevalence and duration of breastfeeding in rural Mexico. *Studies in Family Planning* 18(6):309-319.

Prentice, A.M.
1983   Prenatal dietary supplementation of African women and birth-weight. *Lancet* 489-
         492.
Prentice, A.M., T.J. Cole, F.A. Foord, W.H. Lamb, and R.G. Whitehead
1987   Increased birthweight after prenatal dietary supplementation of rural African women.
         American Journal of Clinical Nutrition 46:912-925.
Pringle, G., and Y.G. Matola
1967   *Report on The Pare-Taveta Vital Statistics Survey, 1962-1966.* Nairobi: East
         African Common Services Organization.
Programme for Control of Acute Respiratory Infections
1990   *Acute Respiratory Infections in Children: Case Management in Small Hospitals in
         Developing Countries.* WHO/ARI/190.5. Geneva: World Health Organization.
Programme for Control of Diarrhoeal Diseases
1991a   International differences in clinical patterns of diarrhoeal deaths: a comparison of
         children from Brazil, Senegal, Bangladesh, and India. Unpublished report. World
         Health Organization.
1991b   Interim Programme Report 1990. World Health Organization.
Puffer, R., and C. Serrano
1973   *Patterns of Mortality in Childhood.* Pan American Health Organization Scientific
         Publication No. 262. Washington, D.C.: Pan American Health Organization.
Rahaman, M.M., K.M.S. Aziz, Y. Patwari, and M.H. Munshi
1979   Diarrhoeal mortality in two Bangladeshi villages with and without community-
         based oral rehydration therapy. *Lancet* 809-812.
Rahaman, M.M., K.M.S. Aziz, M.H. Munshi, Y. Patwari, and M. Rahman
1982   A diarrhea clinic in rural Bangladesh: Influence of distance, age, and sex on
         attendance and diarrheal mortality. *American Journal of Public Health* 72:1124-
         1128.
Rahmathullah, L., B.A. Underwood, R.D. Thulasiraj, R.C. Milton, K. Ramaswamy, R. Rahmathullah,
and G. Babu
1990   Reduced mortality among children in southern India receiving a small weekly dose
         of vitamin A. *New England Journal of Medicine* 323(14):929-934.
Rashad, H.
1989   Oral rehydration therapy and its effect on child mortality in Egypt. *Journal of
         Biosocial Science* (supplement 10):105-114.
1992   The mortality impact of oral rehydration therapy in Egypt: Re-appraisal of evi-
         dence. Pp. 135-160 in K. Hill, ed., *Child Health Priorities for the 1990s.* Balti-
         more, Md.: The Johns Hopkins University Institute for International Programs.
Rebiere, I., D. Lévy-Bruhl, and V. Goulet
1990   Estimation de l'efficacité de la vaccination anti-rougeoleuse à partir de l'enquête
         nationale d'évaluation de la couverture vaccinale menée en 1989, en milieu scolaire.
         Bulletin Epidemiologique Hebdomadaire 38:165.
Reddy, V., P. Bhaskaram, N. Raghuramulu, R.C. Milton, V. Rao, J. Madhusudan, and K.V.R.
Krishna
1986   Relationship between measles, malnutrition, and blindness: A prospective study
         of Indian children. *American Journal of Clinical Nutrition* 44:924-930.
Republique du Burundi
1993   *Bulletin Epidiologique du Burundi* 1(1):16.
Rieder, H.L.
1992   Interventions to reduce childhood morbidity and mortality from tuberculosis. In
         K. Hill, ed., *Child Health Priorities for the 1990s.* Baltimore, Md.: The Johns
         Hopkins University Institute for International Programs.

Roberts, S.B., A.A. Paul, T.J. Cole, and R.G. Whitehead
   1982   Seasonal changes in activity, birth weight and lactational performance in rural Gambian women. *Transactions of the Royal Society of Tropical Medicine and Hygiene* 76:668-678.

Robertson, R.L., S.O. Foster, H.F. Hull, and P.J. Williams
   1985   Cost-effectiveness of immunization in the Gambia. *Journal of Tropical Medicine Hygiene* 88(5):343-351.

Rodrigues, L.C.
   1991   EPI target diseases: Measles, tetanus, polio, tuberculosis, pertussis, and diphtheria. Pp. 173-189 in R.G. Feachem and D.T. Jamison, eds., *Disease and Mortality in Sub-Saharan Africa.* New York: Oxford University Press for The World Bank.

Rosenzweig, M.R., and T.P. Schultz
   1983   Estimating a household production function: Heterogeneity, the demand for helath inputs, and their effects on birth weight. *Journal of Political Economy* 91(5):723-746.

Ross, D.E.
   1986   The trained traditional birth attendant and neonatal tetanus. In A.M. Maglacas and J. Simons, eds., *The Potential of the Traditional Birth Attendant.* WHO Offset Publication No. 95. Geneva: World Health Organization.

Rowland, M.G.M., T.J. Cole, and R.G. Whitehead
   1977   A quantitative study into the role of infection in determining nutritional status in Gambian village children. *British Journal of Nutrition* 37:441-450.

Rowland, M.G.M., R.A.E. Barrell, and R.G. Whitehead
   1978   Bacterial contamination in traditional Gambian weaning foods. *Lancet* 136-138.

Rowland, M.G., S.G. Goh-Rowland, and T.J. Cole
   1988   Impact of infection on the growth of children from 0 to 2 years in an urban West African community. *American Journal of Clinical Nutrition* 47:134-138.

Rozendaal, J.A.
   1989   Impregnated mosquito nets and curtains for self-protection and vector control. *Tropical Diseases Bulletin* 86(supplement) R1-441.

Sazawal, S., and R.E. Black
   1992   Meta-analysis of intervention trials evaluating case management of pneumonia in community settings: An appraisal of the impact on infant and child mortality. *Lancet* 340(ii):528-533.

Schofield, F.D., V.M. Tucker, and G.R. Westbrook
   1961   Neonatal tetanus in New Guinea: Effect of active immunization in pregnancy. *British Medical Journal* 2:785-789.

Schultz, T.P.
   1984   Studying the impact of household economic and community variagles on child mortality. Pp. 215-236 in W.H. Mosley and L.C. Chen, eds., *Child Survival: Strategies for Research. Population and Development Review* supplement to volume 10. New York: Population Council.

Schulzer, M., J.M. Fitzgerald, D.A. Enarson, and S. Grzybowski
   1992   An estimate of the future size of the tuberculosis problem in sub-Saharan Africa resulting from HIV infection. *Tubercle and Lung Disease* 73:52-58.

Schwoebel V., B. Hubert, and J. Grosset
   1993   Impact of BCG on tuberulous meningitis in France in 1990 [letter]. *Lancet* 340:611.

Scrimshaw, N.S. et al.
   1968   Nutrition and infection field study in Guatemalan villages, 1959-1964. V. Disease incidence among preschool children under natural village conditions, with improved diet and with medical and public health services. *Archives of Environmental Health* 16:223-234.

Segamba, L., V. Ndikumasabo, C. Makinson, and M. Ayad
1988   *Enquête Démographique et de Santé au Burundi.* Gitega, Burundi: Ministère de l'Intérieur; Columbia, Md.: Institute for Resource Development/Westinghouse.

Selwyn, B.J.
1990   The epidemiology of acute respiratory tract infection in young children: Comparison of findings from several developing countries. *Review of Infectious Diseases* 12(8):S870-S888.

Shapiro, S.
1968   *Infant, Perinatal, Maternal and Childhood Mortality in the United States.* Cambridge, Mass.: Harvard University Press.

Smedman, L., G. Sterky, L. Mellander, and S. Wall
1987   Anthropometry and subsequent mortality in groups of children aged 6-59 months in Guinea-Bissau. *American Journal of Clinical Nutrition* 46(2):369-373.

Smith, P.G.
1988   Epidemiological methods to evaluate vaccine efficacy. *British Medical Bulletin* 44(3):679-690.

Snow, R.W., J.R.M. Armstrong, D. Foster, M.T. Winstanley, V.M. Marsh, C.R.J.C. Newton, C. Waruiru, I. Mwangi, P.A. Winstanley, and K. Marsh
1992   Childhood deaths in Africa: Uses and limitations of verbal autopsies. *Lancet* 340(ii):351-355.

Sokal, D.C., G. Imboua-Bogui, G. Soga, C. Emmou, and T.S. Jones
1988   Mortality from neonatal tetanus in rural Côte d'Ivoire. *Bulletin of the World Health Organization* 66(1):69-76.

Sommer, A.
1982   *Nutritional Blindness: Xerophthalmia and Keratomalacia.* New York: Oxford University Press.

Sommer, A., G. Faich, and J. Quesada
1975   Mass distribution of vitamin A and the prevention of keratomalacia. *American Journal of Ophthalmology* (80):1073-1080.

Sommer, A., I. Tarwotjo, E. Djunaedi, K.P. West, A.A. Loeden, R. Tilden, and L. Mele
1986   Impact of vitamin A supplementation on childhood mortality. *Lancet* 1169-1173.

South African Medical Journal
1989   Whooping cough—A neglected disease in southern Africa (letter). *South African Medical Journal* 76(11):634-635.

Spencer, H.C., D.C.O. Kaseje, W.H. Mosley, E.K.N. Sempebwa, A.Y. Huong, and J.M. Roberts
1987   Impact on mortality and fertility of a community-based malaria control programme in Saradidi, Kenya. *Annals of Tropical Medicine and Parasitology* 81(supplement 1):36-45.

Stanfield, J.P., and A. Galazka
1984   Neonatal tetanus in the world today. *Bulletin of the World Health Organization* 62(4):647.

Stanley, S.J., C. Howland, M.M. Stone, and I. Sutherland
1981   BCG vaccination of children against leprosy in Uganda: Final results. *Journal of Hygiene (Cambridge)* 87:233-248.

Stoto, M.A.
1993   Models of the demographic effect of AIDS. In K. Foote, K. Hill, and L. Martin, eds., *Demographic Change in Sub-Saharan Africa.* Panel on the Population Dynamics of Sub-Saharan Africa, Committee on Population. Washington, D.C.: National Academy Press.

Strebel, P., G. Hussey, C. Metcalf, D. Smith, D. Hanslo, and J. Simpson
1991   An outbreak of whooping cough in a highly vaccinated urban community. *Journal of Tropical Pediatrics* 37(2):71-76.
Sudanese Ministry of Health and World Health Organization
1981   *Infant and Early Childhood Mortality in Relation to Fertility Patterns: Report of an Ad-Hoc Survey in Greater Khartoum and in the Blue Nile, Kassala and Kordofan Provinces, 1974-1976.* Khartoum: Ministry of Health; Geneva: World Health Organization.
Sudre, P., G. ten Dam, and A. Kochi
1992   Tuberculosis: A global overview of the situation today. *Bulletin of the World Health Organization* 70(2):149-159.
Susser, M., F. Marolla, and J. Fleiss
1972   Birth weight, fetal age and perinatal mortality. *American Journal of Epidemiology* 96(3):197-204.
Tarwotjo, I., A. Sommer, K. West, Jr., E. Djunaedi, L. Mele, B. Hawkins, and the Aceh Study Group
1987   Influence of participation on mortality in a randomized trial of vitamin A prophylaxis 1-3. *American Journal of Clinical Nutrition* 45:466-471.
Taylor, P., and S.L. Mutambu
1986   A review of the malaria situation in Zimbabwe with special reference to the period 1972-1981. *Transactions of the Royal Society of Tropical Medicine and Hygiene* 80(1):12-19.
Taylor, W.R., R.K. Mambu, M. ma-Disu, and J.M. Weinman
1988   Measles control efforts in urban Africa complicated by high incidence of measles in the first year of life. *American Journal of Epidemiology* 127(4):788-794.
Tekçe, B.
1982   Oral rehydration therapy: An assessment of mortality effects in rural Egypt. *Studies in Family Planning* 13(11):315-327.
Tidjani, O., A. Amedome, and H.G. ten Dam
1986   The protective effect of BCG vaccination of the newborn against childhood tuberculosis in an African community. *Tubercle* 67:269-281.
Tielsch, J.M., K.P. West, J. Katz, M.C. Chirambo, L. Schwab, G.J. Johnson, T. Tizazu, J. Swartwood, and A. Sommer
1986   Prevalence and severity of xerophthalmia in southern Malawi. *American Journal of Epidemiology* 124:561-568.
Tomkins, A.
1981   Nutritional status and severity of diarrhoea among preschool children in rural Nigeria. *Lancet* (i):860-862.
Tomkins, A.M., D.T. Dunn, and R.J. Hayes
1989   Nutritional status and risk of morbidity among young Gambian children allowing for social and environmental factors. *Transactions of the Royal Society of Tropical Medicine and Hygiene* 83:282-287.
Tomkins, A., A. Bradley, A. Bradley-Moore, B. Greenwood, S. MacFarlane, and H. Gilles
1991   Morbidity and mortality at Malumfashi, Nigeria, 1975-79; Studies of child health in Hausaland. In R.G. Feachem and D.T. Jamison, eds., *Disease and Mortality in Sub-Saharan Africa.* New York: Oxford University Press for The World Bank.
Touchette, P.E., J. Elder, and M. Nagiel
1990   How much oral rehydration solution is actually administered during home-based therapy? *Journal of Tropical Medicine and Hygiene* 93:28-34.
Traore, B., M. Konate, and C. Stanton
1989   *Enquête Démographique et de Santé au Mali 1987.* Bamako, Mali: Centre d'Etudes

et de Recherches sur la population pour le Développement; Columbia, Md.: Institute for Resource Development/Westinghouse.

Trape, J.F.
1987   Malaria and urbanization in Central Africa: The example of Brazzaville. Rural areas. Part I: Description of the town and review of previous surveys. *Transactions of the Royal Society of Tropical Medicine and Hygiene* 81(2):1-9.

Trape, J.F., F. Legros, P. Ndiaye, L. Konate, I.B. Bah, S. Diallo, F. Verdier, I. Hatin, and J. Le Bras
1989   Chloroquine-resistant *Plasmodium falciparum* malaria in Senegal. *Transactions of the Royal Society of Tropical Medicine and Hygiene* 83:761.

Tuberculosis Control Programme and Expanded Programme on Immunization
1986   Efficacy of infant BCG immunization. *Weekly Epidemiologic Record* 28(11):216-217.

United Nations
1984   *Child Mortality Estimates: A Data Base for Developing Countries.* New York: United Nations.
1991   *World Population Prospects 1990.* New York: United Nations.
1992   *Child Mortality Estimates: A Data Base for Developing Countries.* New York: United Nations.

United Nations Children's Fund
1991   *The State of the World's Children 1991.* Oxford: Oxford University Press.
1992   Evaluation of growth monitoring and promotion programmes. Workshop report. Nairobi, Kenya.

United Nations Department of International Economic and Social Affairs
1983   *Manual X: Indirect Techniques for Demographic Estimation.* New York: United Nations.

U.S. Agency for International Development
1991   *HIV Infection and AIDS: A Report to Congress on the USAID Program for Prevention and Control.* Washington, D.C.: U.S. Agency for International Development.

University of Zambia, Central Statistical Office, and Institute for Resource Development
1992   *Zambia Demographic and Health Survey 1992 (Preliminary Report).* Lusaka, Zambia: University of Zambia and Central Statistical Office; Columbia, Md.: Institute for Resource Development/Macro International, Inc.

van der Werf, T.S., D.G. Groothuis, and B. van Klingeren
1989   High initial drug resistance in pulmonary tuberculosis in Ghana. *Tubercle* 70:249-255.

van der Werf, G.K. Dade, and T.W. van der Mark
1990   Patient compliance with tuberculosis treatment in Ghana: Factors influencing adherence to therapy in a rural service programme. *Tubercle* 71:247-252.

van Ginneken, J.K., and A.S. Muller
1984   *Maternal and Child Health in Rural Kenya.* London: Croom Helm.

van Lerberghe, W.
1989   *Kasongo: Child Mortality and Growth in a Small African Town.* London: Smith-Gordon.

van Lerberghe, W., and K. Pangu
1988   Comprehensive can be effective: The influence of coverage with a health centre network on the hospitalisation patterns in the rural area of Kasongo, Zaire. *Social Science and Medicine* 26(9):949-955.

Van Steenbergen, W., D.A.A. Mossell, J.A. Kusin, and A.A.J. Jansen
1983   Agents affecting health of mother and children in a rural area of Kenya. *Tropical and Geographic Medicine* 35:193-197.

Velema, J.P., E. Alihonou, T. Gandaho, and F. Hounye
1991   Childhood mortality among users and non-users of primary health care in a rural West African community. *International Journal of Epidemiology* 20(2):474-479.

Vernon, A.A., W.R. Taylor, A. Biey, K.M. Mundeke, A. Chahnazarian, H. Habicht, M. Mutombo, and B. Makani
1993   Changes in use of health services in a rural health zone in Zaire: A public health case study. *International Journal of Epidemiology* (forthcoming).

Victora, C., P. Smith, J. Vaughan, L. Nobre, C. Lombardi, A. Teixeria, S. Fuchs, L. Moreira, L. Gigante, and F. Barros
1988   Influence of birth weight on mortality from infectious diseases: A case-control study. *Pediatrics* 81(6):807-811.

Vijayaraghavan, K., G. Radhaiah, B.S. Prakasam, K.V.R. Sarma, and V. Reddy
1990   Effect of massive dose vitamin A on morbidity and mortality in Indian children. *Lancet* 336:1342-1344.

Walsh, J.A., and K.S. Warren
1979   Selective primary health care: An interim strategy for disease control in developing countries. *New England Journal of Medicine* 301(18):967-974.

Warsame, M., W. Wernsdorfer, M. Willcox, A. Kulane, and J. Bjorkman
1991   The changing pattern of *Plasmodium falciparum* susceptibility to chloroquine but not to mefloquine in a mesoendemic area of Somalia. *Transactions of the Royal Society of Tropical Medicine and Hygiene* 85:200-203.

Wassilak, S., and E. Berlin
1986   Tetanus. In J.M. Last, ed., *Public Health and Preventive Medicine*. Norwalk, Conn.: Appleton-Century-Crofts.

Waterlow, J.C.
1972   Classification and definition of protein-calorie malnutrition. *British Medical Journal* 3(826):566-569.

West, K.P. Jr., R.P. Pokhrel, J. Katz, S.C. LeClerq, S.K. Khatry, S.R. Shrestha, E.K. Pradhan, J.M. Tielsch, M.R. Pandey, and A. Sommer
1991   Efficacy of vitamin A in reducing preschool child mortality in Nepal. *Lancet* 338(8759):67-71.

Weyer, K., and H.H. Kleeberg
1992   Primary and acquired drug resistance in adult black patients with tuberculosis in South Africa: Results of a continuous national drug resistance surveillance programme involvement. *Tubercle and Lung Disease* 73:106-112.

Whittle, H.C., M.G.M. Rowland, W.H. Mann, and R.A. Lewis
1984   Immunisation of 4-6 months-old Gambian infants with Edmonston-Zagreb measles vaccine. *Lancet* (ii):834-837.

Whittle, H.C., G. Mann, M. Eccles, and K. O'Neill
1988   Effects of dose and strain of vaccine on success of measles vaccination of infants aged 4-5 months. *Lancet* (i):963-966.

Working Group on Kenya
1993   *Population Dynamics of Kenya*. Panel on the Population Dynamics of Sub-Saharan Africa, Committee on Population, National Research Council. Washington, D.C.: National Academy Press.

World Bank
1989   *Sub-Saharan Africa: From Crisis to Sustainable Growth*. Washington, D.C.: The World Bank.

World Health Organization
1975   Immunization against whooping cough. *WHO Chronicle* 29:365-367.

1980   The incidence of low birth weight: A critical review of available information. *World Health Statistics Quarterly* 33(3):197-226.

1982   *Chemotherapy of Leprosy Control Programmes.* Technical Report Series No. 675. Geneva: World Health Organization.

1984   *Malaria Control as Part of Primary Health Care.* Technical Report Series 712. Geneva: World Health Organization.

1985   *World Health Organization Demographic Yearbook.* Geneva: World Health Organization.

1988   Impact of oral rehydration therapy on hospital admissions and case-fatality rates for diarrheal disease: Results from 11 countries. *Weekly Epidemiological Record* 8:49-52.

1990   *A Vision for the World: Global Elimination of Neonatal Tetanus by the Year 1995. Plan of Action.* Geneva: World Health Organization.

World Health Organization Scientific Group on the Chemotherapy of Malaria

1990   *Practical Chemotherapy of Malaria.* Technical Report Series No. 805. Geneva: World Health Organization.

Wright, E.A.

1990   Low birthweight in the Plateau Region of Nigeria. *East African Medical Journal* 67(12):894-899.

Zeitlin, M.F.

1981   Upper Volta case study of home-based community-level weaning food development. Pp. 79-167 in J. Heimendinger, M.F. Zeitlin, and J.E. Austin, eds., *Nutrition Intervention in Developing Countries, Study IV. Formulated Foods, Study IV.* Cambridge, Mass.: Oelgeschlager, Gunn & Hain.

Zimbabwe Central Statistical Office and Institute for Resource Development

1989   *Zimbabwe Demographic and Health Survey 1988.* Harare, Zimbabwe: Central Statistical Office; Columbia, Md.: Institute for Resource Development/Macro Systems, Inc.

Zumrawi, F.Y., H. Dimond, and J.C. Waterlow

1987   Effects of infection on growth in Sudanese children. *Human Nutrition: Clinical Nutrition* (41C):453-461.